SPOILING CHILDHOOD

SPOILING CHILDHOOD

How Well-Meaning Parents
Are Giving Children Too Much—
But Not What They Need

. . . . . .

DIANE EHRENSAFT, PhD

Foreword by Lillian B. Rubin, PhD

THE GUILFORD PRESS
New York   London

© 1997 The Guilford Press
A Division of Guilford Publications, Inc.
72 Spring Street, New York, NY 10012

Printed in the United States of America

This book is printed on acid-free paper.

Last digit is print number: 9 8 7 6 5 4 3 2 1

Library of Congress Cataloging-in-Publication Data

Ehrensaft, Diane.
    Spoiling childhood: how well-meaning parents are giving
  children too much—but not what they need / Diane Ehrensaft.
        p. cm.
    Includes bibliographical references and index.
    ISBN 1-57230-211-9
    1. Child rearing. 2. Parenting. 3. Parent and child.
  I. Title.
  HQ769.E513 1997
  649'.1—dc21   97-13797
                                                          CIP

*This book is dedicated
to the memory of Peter K. Hawley,
a wonderful father to a father.*

Acknowledgments

It is difficult to pay tribute to all the people who have helped make this book possible, because much of what I have learned about parents and children has come from the great fortune of having so many wonderful families around me. So I want to begin by giving thanks to all the parents who have shared their lives with me, either through research interviews, clinical consultations, personal friendships, or collegial conversations. I feel even more indebted to the children I have come to know over the course of creating this book—children who have come to me for therapy, my own children's friends, my relatives who are small, and the children who have been part of my "fictive" extended family for so many years.

To the specific people who have helped me write this book, I first want to thank Barbara Waterman for her very careful and thoughtful readings of drafts, along with our many long discussions over sushi about children and self-development. Marcy Whitebook, in addition to bringing her expertise as a mother and as a developmental and child care expert to her comments on my manuscripts, has been an inspirational source, long-time close friend, and comrade since we first worked together in The Children's Group in 1973. Ronald Elson has been not only a warm and sympathetic reader with a father's and psychiatrist's critical eye, but also a walking testimonial and learning experience for me about the possibility of being a wonderful parent in harried times, which is what this book is all about. Anne Bernstein has been especially important to me, not just as a clear and lucid reader and editor of my work, but also as a close colleague and intimate personal friend who has taught me so much about thinking not just about the child, but the child as part of a family. Gail Kaufman, one of my very closest comrades in motherhood, has also been my mentor in teaching me that a book is not just to be written but also to be read.

One person in particular needs thanks in so many directions that it is hard to know where to start. Lillian Rubin is not only the writer of the Foreword of this book, but the person who supports me the most, challenges me the most, and holds me to the highest standard of craft, matched only by the one she sets for herself. She has read every word of every draft of this book, and she is the close and wonderful, friend, editor, and critic that every person should be so lucky to have while writing a book, and every other moment, too.

There is also another group of people who have been an inspiration to me and a source of great knowledge and wisdom about parents and children; they are the people with whom I have shared my child clinical work over the past decades. My utmost gratitude goes to Gloria Lawrence, for her humor, dedication, and weekly shared insights into the lives of the children and families she works with, and to my child consultation group—Victor Bonfilio, Eileen Keller, Joan Pechanec, Bonnie Rottier, and Stephen Walrod—without whom I would never know all that I know about the inner lives of children and the parents who raise them.

My editor at The Guilford Press, Kitty Moore, has been my strongest advocate in writing this book. She pushed and pushed me until she thought I had finally got it right, and all the while with great warmth, clarity, and conviction. She is the editor we all dream of having, and I thank her for being that person—present, persistent, wise, and empathic.

I have saved the most important acknowledgments for last. First, to my daughter, Rebecca Ehrensaft-Hawley, and my son, Jesse Ehrensaft-Hawley—there is no way to express the depth of my gratitude for their love and laughter and for teaching me that it is truly possible to raise two wonderful human beings despite all our foibles. And finally, to their father, my husband, Jim Hawley, who has not only read and critiqued draft after draft of this book, but has been there for me through every up, every down, and every middle of the night obsession that is my wont, both in writing and in life. There is no one who could be a better role model of the good-enough father, and as my partner in parenting, he has shared with me the gift of experiencing how truly wonderful raising a child can be.

Foreword

"Who will raise the children?" That's the question Americans have been asking fretfully since increasing numbers of women have entered the labor force. Now Diane Ehrensaft has given us the answer. Parents are raising their children, just as they always have. The question, she insists, is not *who* is raising the children but *how* they are being raised.

Are today's mothers and fathers the narcissistic, self-centered parents some experts denounce? Or are they the overly concerned, overindulgent parents that periodically claim media attention? Neither and both, says Dr. Ehrensaft in this complex, wide-ranging, and fascinating analysis of the problems of parenting in the 1990s.

The questions may be framed differently, but the issue of how we raise our children has preoccupied Americans for most of this century. In the years before World War II, children were widely seen as a bundle of id impulses awaiting parental and social control. Advice manuals were largely concerned with behavior, offering parents instruction on how to mold a child to fit the social norms of the day. It was an adult-centered world that children of that era entered, and they were expected to take their place in it without causing too many ripples in the lives or the environment of those who controlled it. This meant that there was a relatively rigid and straightforward set of rules and expectations, ranging from when an infant would eat, sleep, and be toilet trained to when and how a small child was permitted to speak in the presence of adults.

• • •

The years following World War II saw a distinct softening in our view of childhood. Instead of focusing on controlling children, psychologists began to think about their development, about what it was possible to expect of a child at each age and stage of those early years. The result was the emergence of modern theories of child development—theories that traced the physiological and neurological developmental processes of infancy and early childhood with the same precision with which geographers map the physical terrain.

It wasn't long before advice books were telling mothers and fathers exactly what to expect at each developmental stage. Parents anxiously scanned the pages of Arnold Gessell and Frances Ilg's bestselling *Child Development*,[1] checking to see if the baby smiled on cue, turned over, sat up, walked, spoke at the "right" time. Mothers, nearly universally the primary caretakers of the children, traded stories wherever they met, always looking for reassurance that their child's development matched the newly established norms.

It was a small step from worrying about their children's physical and neurological development to their psychological well-being. Soon the man who would become the nation's baby doctor, Benjamin Spock, was advising parents on all manner of issues, from how to recognize a measles rash to the necessity for care in dealing with a child's tender psyche. Resting his case on the new developmental theories, he cautioned parents that children were threatened with psychological damage if parental expectations exceeded a child's capabilities.

Now, instead of entering an adult-centered world, children became the center of family life and concerns. It was the child whose world was protected from intrusion; the child, not the parent, who took control of when she would eat, sleep, go to the toilet. Whereas in earlier years children were expected to be seen but not heard, these parents often stood mute while their offspring were both seen and heard. Almost overnight, it seemed, we went from the injunction that we risked spoiling the child if we spared the rod to the fear that using the rod—or its verbal disciplinary equivalent—would crush the child. Permissiveness became the order of the day.

It was during this time, in the early 1950s, that I had my first experience with what could happen when this new permissiveness was taken to the extreme. I was visiting a friend, chatting comfortably in her kitchen, when her four-year-old, who had been sleeping, entered the room and demanded her attention. When she didn't respond instantly, he ran up and began to hit her, his little fists pummeling her face and breasts as she tried quietly to calm him. But he would not be soothed. Instead, his rage out of control, he rushed to the kitchen counter, picked up a knife that lay there, and threw it across the room, narrowly missing my ear. First I was stunned, then furious. But my friend gently gathered her son up in her arms and, without a word of reprimand, explained, "He's just jealous because you're here. He doesn't like it when I'm not giving him all my attention."

The age of permissiveness flowed almost naturally into the children's rights movement. As liberation movements proliferated during the 1960s and 1970s, children joined the list of the oppressed, put there by advocates who asserted that children were little people who had been deprived of a voice in their own destiny. Now the fragile child who needed constant care and attention—the child who would be, in the language of 1950s child rearing, "traumatized" by the wrong or thoughtless deed—was joined by the child as knowing actor. In this view, the child deserved equal standing in the social world; adult rules and boundaries were unnecessary infringements on the child's liberty.

Extreme, perhaps, but an idea that, in a more modified form, has become sufficiently diffused into the culture of parenthood so that all too many parents no longer feel free to tell a child what to do. Instead, they engage in what one writer calls a "tot-level Socratic dialogue" that starts with the abnegation of parental authority, whether about when the child should go to bed to whether he would go to school on any given day. "All right, you tell me what *you* think you should do," a parent now asks, praying that the child will come up with the "right" answer.

For fifty years, then, we have been moving toward what Dr. Ehrensaft calls the parenthood crisis—a crisis, she tells us, born of the confused and contradictory definitions of childhood, of our inability to decide whether our children are simply short adults waiting to grow as tall as we are or whether they are innocent, dependent babes who need our constant care and protection.

Unable to settle the question, we have, as she elaborates so brilliantly, merged the two competing visions into one and brought forth the "kinderdult"—her evocative word for childhood's double exposure, the child as half baby/half adult that now dominates the view of childhood held by both parents and professionals alike. The result, she shows us with compelling clarity, is a generation of confused, guilt-ridden parents who pamper and hover over their children at the same time that they permit, even encourage, them to "handle complicated decisions or tasks that might tax even a thirty-year-old."

In story after story taken from her many years of practice as a child psychologist, she provides evidence of the cost to children when parents treat them one moment as tender infants and the next as capable adults. As one troubled eight-year-old patient said, after begging her to tell his parents he isn't a baby, "But could you also tell them to stop talking to me like I'm twenty or something."

In this wise and wonderful book Dr. Ehrensaft tells parents just that—and a lot more. But while any reader, whether parent or professional, will find a wealth of sensitive and intelligent advice on its pages, this is much more than an ordinary "how to" book. For unlike so many "experts" who see families as if they were atoms floating in space, unconnected to the social and institutional world in which they are embedded, Dr. Ehrensaft understands fully the interrelatedness of family and social life.

She abjures the harsh and critical voices that shout so loudly about the failure of family values and that decry the lack of discipline in child rearing, bringing to the discourse instead an informed and compassionate understanding of the social context of family life and the psychological consequences that flow from that. She knows, for example, that when parents are both at work all day, they are likely to feel guilty about what they are not giving their children. And she knows, too, that guilt leads them to overcompensate, often in ways that are damaging to the child.

She knows, also, that the increasing stress in the social and economic world—the fear that there is neither safety nor security in the future—has left parents more uncertain than ever before about what they can do for their children today to ensure that they will have a better tomorrow. And she understands that it's this anxiety that generates the kind of excesses that lead parents to try to ensure, even before the child is born, that he or she will have every competitive advantage.

In chapter after chapter, Dr. Ehrensaft takes up the issues every parent faces: How do we separate our own needs from those of our children? How can we ensure our children's happiness and success? What are age-appropriate behavioral expectations? When do we gratify a child's desires? When do we say no, and how do we make it stick? How can we raise children who freely offer us not just their love, but their respect as well?

Spoiling Childhood is a book that both parents and professionals will turn to eagerly and often. Its pages are filled with delightful, funny, sad real-life stories about children and their parents, about the difficulties we all face today as we try to find ways to bring up our children in a rapidly changing world. Without sacrificing analytic rigor, Diane Ehrensaft raises her humane, thoughtful, and always good-humored voice to point the direction. In doing so, she not only teaches us how to parent more effectively, she also offers an illuminating analysis that explains us to ourselves.

LILLIAN B. RUBIN, PhD
San Francisco, California

Contents

CHAPTER ONE
The Perils of Parenting
1

CHAPTER TWO
Your Majesty, the Baby
23

CHAPTER THREE
And Baby Makes Three, or Is Baby Me?
46

CHAPTER FOUR
Parenting by Guilt
74

CHAPTER FIVE
My Toddler, the Doctor
93

CHAPTER SIX
Pampering Our Children toward Success
121

Contents

• • •

CHAPTER SEVEN
Parents Bartering for Love
151

CHAPTER EIGHT
Use the Rod, Lose the Child
178

CHAPTER NINE
The Kinderdult
207

CHAPTER TEN
Unspoiling Childhood
231

Notes
245

Index
257

SPOILING CHILDHOOD

CHAPTER ONE
• • • • • •

The Perils of Parenting

*Most of us with young children are from a
generation that overthinks, overreacts and
over-analyzes. . . . And we got it in our heads that
not only could we be perfect parents, we must
be. . . . I don't know about you, but I'm ready to
rejoin Planet Earth.*

—JOAN RYAN[1]

My first impulse to write *Spoiling Childhood* was sparked in an
unsuspecting moment while having dinner at our friends' house.
Their five-year-old, a child born to older parents, was racing around
the dining room table on her Big Wheel. I could not hear myself
think, let alone hear the conversation around the table, among both
the adults and the older children assembled. I wondered, "Why do
they let Miranda do this? Isn't someone going to ask her to stop?"
Nobody did. I finally did, as her mother and father looked askance.
I gently suggested to Miranda that she find something a little quieter
to do so we could hear each other talk. She chose the rocking horse
with the screeching springs, set right at the corner of the table. I
surrendered. Later I mused, "Who is this child to my friends that
they live their lives this way, trapped in a child-generated noise
tunnel? In every other way they are sensible people. Why are they
letting their child, a lovely little girl, give us all such a headache?"
My question awakened in me the realization that something profound was occurring in our culture that needed explanation. I felt
driven to find out what it is that governs our parenting today and
why it looks so askew. How can we fix whatever needs to be fixed?

1

I was not satisfied with the explanation for today's out-of-balance parenting being put forth to the American public. Shortly before his death, Bruno Bettelheim, the noted child psychoanalyst, stated, "I think there is a very self-centered generation growing up because parents don't give enough of themselves to their children—not just their time, but their emotions. Like their own parents, they're [the children are] self-centered."[2] Yet listen carefully to the words of one of those "self-centered" parents, a single working mother with a small child: "When I first went back to work, I used to count the hours Rachel and I actually spent together, as if I'd hit upon the magic number that would make everything all right. On the way home from the office, I would panic whenever the train made an unscheduled stop between stations. That meant I would have even less time with my daughter."[3] Hardly enraptured by the time away from her child, this parent is tormented not about what she *will not* give, but what she *cannot* give to her child—more of herself.

Something is wrong with the portrayal of the self-centered parent. As a parent myself, this label offended me—it felt unfair to Rachel's mother and to me and to the parents around me. So what is a more accurate picture of today's parent? I undertook a quest to find out.

THE PARADOX OF PARENTING

Parents today are tagged as a generation preoccupied with work and themselves yet at the same time overly focused on their children. Professionals, policy makers, media critics, and experts of all kinds simultaneously label mothers and fathers as self-indulgent and over-indulgent, as absent and hovering, irresponsible and overcommitted, ill-informed and overeducated.

On the other hand, parents are chastised for putting their own happiness, interests, or achievement first and their children's second, or not at all. The increasing number of hours parents spend away from their children, most often at the workplace, serves as evidence that parents are putting their own work needs and personal activities ahead of time with their sons and daughters. The freedom with which they divorce, with no apparent regard for the children's best interests, is further testimony of their self-involvement. Too preoccupied with themselves, parents ignore the children and let them run wild, creating a generation of hellions and lost souls.

Just as more and more women with children under five have entered the work force, reports are disseminated implying mothers may permanently damage their infants and young children by their absence. Similarly, at the same time that educational budgets are being cut drastically, we hear that academic success is correlated with *parents'*, not schools', involvement in their children's studies and that most parents are not around enough to provide this support.

But then the critics turn around and tell the parents, specifically the middle-class ones, "Your real problem is that you are overindulgent with your children. You spoil them. You shower them with material goods, grant their every passing whim, never say no, and send them to fancy schools, even if you cannot afford it." In that light, modern parents are characterized as hovering caregivers who fawn over, cater to, and dote on their children in a manner heretofore never seen—young Miranda on her Big Wheel. Parents offer friendship instead of guidance. They treat their children likes princes and princesses and prime them for success even before they exit the birth canal.

Years as a child clinician tell me that the results of such indulgence are as dire for the children as the consequences of parental self-involvement. Children become overly self-aggrandized, with a sense of entitlement that makes it difficult for them to live cooperatively in a world of peers. They never learn the meaning of the word "no." They are pressured and pushed, feeling they always have to accomplish for their parents' pleasure. They have a false sense of independence and autonomy. They are never happy unless the focus is on themselves. They lack empathy for others. They will be thwarted in their later intimate relationships and will never develop an authentic sense of self. They are at risk for becoming narcissists.

So I stop and ask the most puzzling question confronting us about parents today. *How could this same group of parents be simultaneously accused of being the most self-centered and self-indulgent, and*

*also the most child-centered and overly indulgent generation of
parents in modern history? Can it be both ways?*

Actually, it can and it is. That is the paradox this book seeks to
explain. In a myriad of ways, we will see how we are a generation
of self-involved parents, with a great deal of weight placed on our
own personal happiness. Yet we are also a generation with a
tremendous investment in being good parents, who go overboard to
provide what we think will be the best for our children. It is this
lethal combination that puts us at risk for spoiling childhood.

Just exactly who is the "we" to whom I refer? *Spoiling Childhood*
is the story of educated, middle-class parents born in the aftermath
of World War II. It is the story of professionals who are highly
invested in both their careers and their families. It includes the people
who read a lot of books about raising children and even some who
write the books themselves.

It is the story of a group of people taking great pains to be good
parents, a group of people who want to parent well but find precious
little time in which to do it. Like the mother on the train, they rush
back and forth between work and home. They are constantly
seesawing between feeling like superparents and like abject failures.
Their story can be a wake-up call to all of us as we approach the
twenty-first century, for it is not just parents without resources, but
also parents with good education, financial resources, and high
motivation who are having a very rough time trying to raise their
children in a reasonable way.

THE CONFUSED PARENT

At ten years old, Jeremy, small in stature, with sparkling eyes and a
cherubic smile, is precocious, unusually bright, and most eloquent.
He's used to saying whatever he wants whenever he wants. To
Jeremy, the phrase "Don't interrupt" might as well be in a foreign
language. He demands his own way and usually gets it. His mother,
with the coaching of her new husband, a seasoned parent himself,
has reached her limit. Here they are, a mile from home, and Jeremy
stalwartly refuses to get back in the car after a shopping expedition.
Mom gives him one warning, spelling out the consequences. Jeremy

takes no heed. Mother and Greg, the stepfather, resolutely drive away, leaving Jeremy, dumbfounded, facing the long walk home.

Jeremy reports to me his prison march, blurting out, "My mother is the meanest mother in the world. I wish I had you for a mother—you're so nice." I ask him, "Jeremy, if you were a parent, what would you do in the same situation?" Without a moment's reflection, the solution comes: "Greg should throw me in the trunk and beat me."

Jeremy, his mother, and Greg are just three people trying to find their way through Jeremy's childhood. They illustrate the confusion and lack of sure footing that plague parents today as they raise their children. They also alert those of us in the profession of child and family mental health to a situation we can no longer deny: Parenthood is in a state of crisis.

Today's mothers and fathers, pegged as both self-centered and overindulgent, may well go down in history as the most maligned generation of parents. It is an undeserved reputation. We are not, any more than mothers and fathers of past generations, bad or selfish parents. More aptly, like Jeremy's mother and stepfather, we are *confused* parents. We live in a moment of history when family life is in rapid flux. In less than one generation, the modern nuclear family—father as breadwinner, mother as homemaker—plummeted from being the dominant household form to a rather small minority of American homes. Both mothers and fathers now go off to work each morning for long hours of the day. Some families have no fathers, others no mothers.

We face a daunting task. We find ourselves raising the next generation within a set of rapidly changing conditions, both at home and outside our front door, that do not lend themselves to successful child rearing. The structure of the workplace; the radical changes in family life; the increasing unpredictability of the environmental, social, and political world; and the sensibilities of a society that puts profit first and families last all have had a deep psychological effect on the men and women who conceive and raise children today.

Along with the harsh social realities confronting them, parents bring their own conflicts, anxieties, attitudes, and emotions into their experience of raising children. Their personal psychology and the social conditions surrounding them get entangled with each other to make successful parenting a Herculean task done against great odds. As we struggle with the challenges of raising our own sons and daughters, we fail to recognize that the problem goes far beyond our personal parenting crises to the culture at large. As a society, we feel out of balance as nurturers of the next generation and have lost our bearings about the goals for children and the means for reaching them. Nobody seems to be clear about whether we want strong-minded individuals or cooperative team players for our next generation. And nobody seems to be clear about how to achieve either one—through gentle love or tough love, freedom or structure, rewards or punishments.

We could say that parenting always comes with problems, but the specific challenges that face the parents of the 1990s existed neither for their mothers or fathers nor for their parents before them. American parents in the 1930s had to sustain the economic blows of the Great Depression. Mothers and fathers in the 1940s faced a major world war, the exodus of men to the battlefield and entrance of women into wartime jobs, and then the return of the men home and the women to the hearth in the aftermath of the war. Parents in the 1950s were met with the glorification of the modern nuclear family and the myth of the ideal parenting partnership—Mom at home, Dad at the workplace. They were also confronted with cold war fears that they and their children might be decimated by a mushroom-shaped cloud. But in each of those three decades there was a dominant directive about raising children, whether it be the advocacy of habit training in the 1930s or the more permissive approaches to child rearing promoted by Benjamin Spock in the 1940s and 1950s.

Today, no such clear directives exist. We have a generation of parents where Mom is expected to be at the workplace, but also at home; where Dad is supposed to strive for accomplishment in work, but also be a nurturing father; where the family two people create may barely resemble the one their children exit. With the dramatic shifts in social conditions and family structures, the people who are supposed to be the experts cannot even agree among themselves on how the children of these parents should be raised. So mothers and fathers find no clear guidelines to shepherd them through the child-rearing years. Instead, they desperately flip-flop from one approach to another—permissive to authoritative, democratic to autocratic, indulgent to withholding.

On a day-to-day level, we float from one dilemma to the next trying to meet our children's needs and construct a workable family life. A divorced mother of a seventeen-year-old has "lost control" of her daughter. Alexis wants the freedom but none of the responsibilities of adulthood—to take an allowance, come and go as she pleases, take food from the refrigerator, but pitch in at home only if she feels like it. Her living quarters would readily be condemned by the local health department. Cynthia Adams, Alexis's mother, is furious at her daughter, yet fears that if she makes any demands on her, Alexis will reject her, maybe even run away. Meanwhile, her next door neighbor, Byron Smith, indulges seven-year-old Sammy's every whim to compensate for his long business meetings away from home, then asks Sammy to act like a man in his absence. And the Smiths' relatives across town bought early phonics flash cards for their preschooler in a concerted effort to accelerate her development, only to read an article warning that such early intervention may put their child at risk for anxiety disorders by middle childhood.

Cynthia Adams, Byron Smith, and his relatives across town are running in circles—they do not have a set of reasonable child-rearing guidelines to inform them, they are stretched too thin between home and work, they make desperate attempts to cater to both themselves and their children. They are not unique. After listening to the plights of mothers and fathers in my consultation room and in my interviews with men and women who share the care of their children, observing and interacting with parents in the community, following the media, reading in scholarly journals, as well as living through my own experience as a mother of this generation, I felt it was time to address parents' angst and confusion, make sense of it, offer parents a way out of their parenting morass, and prescribe possible remedies to the paradox of self-indulgent/overindulgent parenting.

In the midst of working on *Spoiling Childhood*, a mother in a parent workshop I was conducting stood up and asked imploringly, "Could you please tell me *why* our generation is so insecure about parenting and what we're supposed to do about it?" I hope this book will offer an answer to her question, for all of us.

PARENTHOOD AS NEVER BEFORE

November 1981. I come home exhausted. I have just worked a ten-hour day, something I hate but am forced to do occasionally. I'm supposed to go to an important work meeting the next day. My daughter wants to show me her new dance routine. My son is down in the dumps because of a conflict between him and his two best kindergarten friends. He's presently the odd man out, because they like horses more than he does. Tomorrow, I discover belatedly, is my daughter's "authors' day" at school. Parents are invited to come peruse their children's literary creations. My daughter really wants me to be there. So do I. I have a patient who may need to be hospitalized that night. I don't know how I'm going to take care of everything and everyone. I feel like crying. I do.

No Time to Parent

My tears stem from the first of the four major structural factors that make the phenomenon of parenting both remarkable and torturous for parents today: The time to parent has been cut drastically. Despite earlier predictions that America was moving into a period of more leisure time and shorter work weeks, work time in America has been increasing over the last twenty years. In this same period, the participation of middle-class women with children in the workplace has risen dramatically.[4] Yet parents are still straddled with the same responsibilities for raising children as their mothers and fathers before them. Extended families are rarely available to pick up the slack, either because of physical distance or because grandmothers and grandfathers themselves are part of the full-time work force. Like me and the mother who counted the number of train stops on the way home to see her daughter, we are constantly breathless in our desperate efforts to scoop out time and energy for our families and children, when hardly any of either is left in the pot.

It may be true that we are raising a generation of hurried children who are rushed from day care to school to day care or from one activity to another. But it's equally true that we are a generation of hurried parents, pressed to parent perfectly but with precious little time in which to do it. To assuage parents who must simultaneously work for a living and raise children—the vast majority of both mothers and fathers today—we have capitalized on the concept of "quality time": The *amount* of time we spend does not matter as long as it is "good" time. But the sad reality remains that there is simply not much time to be had with the children. We feel little option but to raise our children in a hurried, if not haphazard, fashion.

Fear for Our Children's Future

The second critical factor facing parents is that they no longer have confidence that their children have a good life ahead of them or even right in front of them. The post-World War II life of the 1940s was one that promised prosperity and unlimited opportunity to the young mothers and fathers of that era, an expectation that was passed on to their children. Indeed, those children's growing years were a time of affluence, a time of economic growth, a time when hard work, and not such hard work, could breed success. More young adults went to college than ever before, not just in sheer numbers, but as a percentage of the total population.

Those children have now come of age themselves, only to find that the promise was a false one. As we traverse the last decade of the twentieth century, the future does not look so sanguine. Our city streets are filled with homeless people. Grown children cannot achieve the same standard of living as their parents.[5] We are scared for our children. We have lost confidence that we can deliver to them a better world. And our confidence is further shaken when we look at the world the children live in right now, where government programs for children only continue to disappear, the quality of public education deteriorates, adequate day care is sparse, violence escalates, and growing rates of suicide among American youth tell us that death knocks not only at the door of the old.

Martin is sitting in my office wringing his hands. He has a fifteen-year-old daughter, who is an above-average but not highly motivated student. He himself is a successful lawyer. He has just had lunch with an old law school friend whose daughter graduated with honors in

English from a top university and spent two years trying to find a junior editing job, only to give up and take a job as a secretary. His other friend's son has moved back in with his parents after finishing college because he cannot afford to live on his own with his present wages. Martin is tearful. He has always encouraged his daughter to reach for the stars, but now he fears she won't ever get off the ground.

The children worry, too, not so much about their future but about their lives right now. Gretchen is a teenager I first saw in therapy when she was seven. She was brought by her parents because of an anxiety disorder. Overcoming her problems, she went on to have a happy and fulfilling middle childhood and early adolescence. She was now attending a large public high school and doing well, until a close friend of hers was shot and killed accidentally by another friend who was playing with his father's gun. Gretchen came to see me, again riddled with anxiety. Although her friend's death was the precipitating event, she spilled out tales about people in her high school who had attempted suicide, acquaintances who were strung out on drugs, teenagers whose parents had thrown them out of the house, a teacher who threw a pen at her face. She had apprised her parents, too, of all that she was telling me. They were ruefully aware that their middle-class status in no way shielded their daughter from the worsening conditions for children today.

Fragile Family Ties

Such worry is exacerbated by the third factor impinging on parents today: Children are often the only reliable connection adults now have in their family life. It is a rare bride or groom who genuinely believes the vow " 'Til death do us part," when close to fifty percent of wedding vows end in separation and divorce. Unlike in the past, children are no longer the glue that holds families together. Many partners with children decide they cannot continue in a marriage that is no longer bringing them fulfillment or basic comfort. For others, a marriage filled with strife or abuse is accurately seen as detrimental to the well-being of the children.

For some parents, their children have always been their only permanent connection. With the stigma of unwed motherhood lifted (despite pressures from the extreme right to the contrary), there are women today who have opted out of a marriage contract or parenting partnership altogether and would rather parent on their own from the start. Others have found themselves in that position without choice or with no better options available, as is true for older single women up against the biological clock of childbearing.

This means that spouses or parenting partners may come and go, or never materialize, but presumably sons and daughters will always be there. We rely on our children even more in the absence of extended families and stable neighborhoods and communities. They provide us with a sense of belonging as an antidote to the increased atomization of daily life in America. As we turn to our children to provide stability and consistency and reassurance that somebody indeed loves us and that we are not alone, we cannot afford to think anything bad could happen to them.

A mother called me to discuss the custody schedule she and her ex-husband had set up for their nine-year-old son. Jordan had been adopted when he was four, in the hopes of saving a failing marriage. His adoption only tore the marriage further apart. Lana, the mother, now had primary custody of Jordan. Many an evening she had called me for guidance in a state of exhaustion, frazzled from trying to balance two jobs and single parenting and filled with bitterness about the breakup of her marriage. At times Jordan's demands could drive her to distraction, to the point of her seeing him as her tormentor. Jordan was leaving in two days for a two-and-a-half-week visit with his grandparents. I mistakenly applauded the two-week respite she would have for herself, a short vacation from the daily hassles of single parenting. Feeling totally misunderstood by me, Lana retorted angrily, "Quite the contrary. I don't know how I'm going to survive without Jordan here. What if something happens to him? He's all I've got going for me. I'm so afraid of the loneliness."

The Peter Pan Syndrome

The last factor confronting parenting today is our own psychology: We are a unique generation in our hesitancy to cross the threshold into adulthood. We suffer from the Peter Pan syndrome—children who never wanted to or never believed they would eventually grow up. We have brought with us a legacy of tension between adulthood and childhood that has come to haunt us throughout our parenting years.

In the original story of Peter Pan by James M. Barrie, Peter in fact had many children, the Lost Boys, who were delivered to him in Never-Never Land in their infancy, unclaimed by their families after falling from their perambulators while their nurses were otherwise engaged. As their "captain," Peter had every intention of fathering the abandoned boys, and imported Wendy from London to be their mother in all the gender stereotypic ways in which females are expected to care for children. But the plan broke down. Peter's notions of child-centered and child-run communal families—where children could do whatever they wanted when they wanted—did not blend well with Wendy's internalized values from proper Victorian society. Wendy returned to her homeland, where she could grow up in proper form, taking the Lost Boys with her, while Peter stubbornly remained in Never-Never Land, where children are free and never grow up.

Like Peter with Wendy, the contemporary Peter Pans also have had a problem: The world they envisioned as youth has little in common with the realities they face as parents in the last decade of the twentieth century, a contrast that to them feels as stark as that between Never-Never Land and Victorian England. A generation that grew up with the promise of an easy ticket to success and happiness, we discover that nothing comes so easily—success, happiness, or stable families—and that there are no free lunches.

Despite our wishes never to grow up, in fact, we did. Alice Kahn, a newspaper columnist in her forties, depicts our present plight: "Around the age when previous generations had to grow up, get a job, get a haircut, my generation hit the late '60s. A reprieve. Whole new opportunities to torture our parents as we moved into our twenties. Jobs were for wage slaves. Growing up was for straights. Haircuts were for plastic people."[6]

The generation that came of age in the 1960s is not the only one to qualify for the Peter Pan syndrome. It equally applies to all the youth following behind them who were influenced by the cultural shifts toward consumerism, personal fulfillment, and immediate gratification. That accounts for most people who find themselves parenting children today. The Peter Pan sensibility may not preclude holding jobs, working hard, and taking on adult responsibilities. Remarkably for the Peter Pan generation, those attributes appear to coexist with the impulse to cling tenaciously to the joys of youth and to the delusional belief that youth runs eternal.

So what happens when the Peter Pans begin having children of their own? According to Kahn, "The party was over. 'Just wait until you have kids,' our parents had said smugly, and now we know why." Our party is indeed over, so what do we face?

CHANGING PARENTHOOD, CHANGING CHILDHOOD

We face a terrain in which children are not only being raised in the midst of a redefinition of parenting. Parents are simultaneously functioning in the midst of a redefinition of *childhood*.

The concept of childhood is decidedly culture bound, varying from epoch to epoch and society to society. The proud image of the African child who by age five has responsibility for her younger siblings while her parents work in the fields diverges greatly from the concept of the American kindergartner who is a latchkey kid, left unattended (neglected) while her parents are away at work. The Victorian child who was to be seen but not heard has nothing in common with the late twentieth-century child who is to be actively listened to by all concerned adults. It only makes sense that as the composition and structure of parenting and of family and social life shift, so, too, will our sense of what a child is.

A mother and father come to my office to consult about their eight-year-old's emotional resistances to school. I learn that Joshua has been told by his parents that President Bush may blow up the world with nuclear weapons. I learn that Joshua's mother suggests that Joshua himself negotiate a cut-rate fee with the school director for his after-school care. I also learn that his mother and father, bolstered by magazine articles and "expert" advice, felt that at four Joshua was emotionally ready to be at the birth of his younger sister. Indeed, he was in attendance at the event. But I also later discover that Joshua's mother does not feel her son can handle having to wait one week for an appointment with me, which he himself had requested. He would feel "ripped off," because when he wants something, he expects it now. These parents allow their child to know nothing of delayed gratification but everything about the dangers of nuclear holocaust.

Joshua's parents are not unique in this perception, and Joshua is presently suffering a confusion of identity because of it. With great composure, this unusually serious-looking child tells me in the first appointment, arranged by his parents, that at age eight he is perfectly capable of handling his worries himself and is in no need of my help, thank you very much. But in the next session, the one that he himself requested, he sits, tense and frightened, his eye twitching and his hands wringing, like a little old man with a baby's face. He has changed his mind, he could use my help, he wants to talk to me in private. He begs me to get his parents to stop hovering over him all the time and to stop thinking he doesn't know how to do anything himself. And then he adds, "But could you also tell them to stop talking to me like I'm twenty or something."

Juliet fully believed her two-year-old daughter, Dorothy, was capable of making her own decisions as to whether she wanted to share her toys with other children or not. But she still spoonfed her daughter. When Dorothy was seven, Juliet never intervened when Dorothy dominated her younger sister or insisted on her way with other children. She believed that children, like adults, have the capabilities to work these things out themselves and should be respectfully left to their own resources. But Juliet never asked Dorothy to do a household chore, because she felt a seven-year-old was far too young to handle such a responsibility.

In one moment we perceive our children as ready to handle complicated decisions or tasks that might tax even a thirty-year-old. Martine tells her three-year-old daughter, Laurel, that *Laurel* should talk to her father to tell him she does not like it when he sleeps without pajamas when she visits his home. The next moment we cannot fathom our children as anywhere but in the cradle, and we worry that if their every passing wish is not granted we will trample on their fragile and infantile constitutions. Martine grants the same little Laurel every one of her three or four screaming requests for baby bottles throughout the night, leaving both mother and daughter hopelessly deprived of sleep.

Some are alarmed that childhood is simply disappearing. Children no longer appear in TV, movies, and even real life stories. Instead, we see images of miniature adults, perhaps etched in our minds most memorably in the smiling face of seven-year-old Jessica Dubroff minutes before her tragic death in a 1996 plane crash, while attempting to set a record as the youngest child to fly solo across the country. Tastes and styles of children and adults are steadily merging. Mother and daughter stroll hand in hand through Greenwich Village in their matching Nikes and designer jeans. Father and son bicker over who has first dibs on the new Rolling Stones tape. On a more somber note, increasing rates of alcoholism, drug use, sexual activity, and crime among the young provide further evidence that childhood is steadily diminishing as a separate category.[7] The trend toward being more and more grown up starts young and keeps progressing. By age two, toddlers often have their own lunch box; by age seven, their own bus pass; and by fourteen, their own condoms.

David Elkind, in his widely read book, *The Hurried Child,*[8] reports that today's children are pressured to achieve, to succeed, to please, to hurry and grow up. Consumed by their own stress and worries, feeling more afraid, alone, and professionally insecure than parents in the past, mothers and fathers attempt to bolster their own self-esteem by having precocious and high-achieving sons and daughters.

A quick sampling of newspaper and magazine accounts over a two-year period, 1987–1988, reveals the following titles: "Super-babies Aren't Happy Babies," "Are Children Now Lacking the Time to Just Be Kids?," "The Superbaby Burnout Syndrome," "The Fuss over the Rushed Child," "Children of Fast-Track Parents," "Kids in the Fast Lane," "Fast Track to Puberty." Scratch the surface and an abundance of such reports spills out, testimony to the fact that not just Elkind, but a growing number of social critics are becoming increasingly alarmed by the perceived dangers to these "children in the fast track." If childhood is truly disappearing, we have good reason to worry—this acceleration of children's developmental processes, left unchecked, can only do harm to their maturation and growth.

Paradoxically, however, at the same time that childhood is disappearing, a multimillion dollar industry has emerged to service it. We have children's toothpaste, children's aerobic equipment, even a children's bank in Manhattan. Marketing experts and advertisers devote inordinate amount of time designing campaigns to appeal to the specialized interests of children. Well before children could ever make purchase choices for themselves, the programming has already begun in infancy, as they are pushed in the high-priced, space-age-designed strollers their parents feel compelled to buy. Presently, big business both designates and reflects the image of the child as a highly complicated being with very separate needs and desires. If childhood was really disappearing, capitalist enterprise would be in for a big loss.

And how could childhood be disappearing when it actually goes on for more years than ever before? Young children may indeed be rushed to learn to read and play piano. But as those same children approach the end of the teen years, no one appears to be in a hurry to push them out of the nest. We may be scurrying our sons and daughters through their growing up years, but then we put a stopper on it when they approach the finish line. In contrast to past generations, childhood dependency today is increasingly prolonged well into young adulthood. Advanced education and training now extend far beyond the high school years for a large number of young men and women, leaving them suspended in a financially dependent status well into the age when their own parents and grandparents had already become mothers and fathers and stable members of the work force. Even for those high school graduates who do not go on for advanced training, the rising costs of living in this country make it near impossible for many young adults to support themselves outside their parents' home.

In reality, it is not simply that children are being rushed or that they are being infantilized. Rushed, hurried "superkids" are only half the picture. The same children who are pushed and hurried about are coddled, protected, and catered to. Not by selfish or uncaring parents, but by *confused* parents who have no clear picture of what a child is and are unconscious of the vacillations between hurrying our children and holding them back. As a result, childhood is simultaneously contracting and expanding in some bizarre fashion.

Parents today are strongly influenced by an image of childhood that is actually a double exposure: the young sophisticate superimposed over the "babe in the woods." This image does not go away, even as our children enter adulthood. I perceive my nineteen-year-old son as quite capable of handling the academic demands of his college. I think he is competent to travel throughout the world on his own. But I have to struggle to remind myself that he is old enough to arrange his own allergy shots or make his own airline reservations or even order his own food in a restaurant.

It's this double exposure—half baby/half adult—that more accurately describes parents' confused perception of their children today. It embodies wild oscillations between the child as a short-standing, autonomous individual moving toward maturity (Joshua who negotiates his own child care fees) and the child as an innocent, dependent, or primitive young thing in need of care and protection (Joshua who must be gratified now). I dub this double exposure the "kinderdult." I believe the kinderdult is the best descriptor of the prevailing vision of children today and that it dominates the thinking and actions of parents and professionals alike. I also believe it is an image that contributes to the spoiling of childhood.

An example comes to mind, involving a controversy among two groups of professionals. In recent years the Board of Education in Palo Alto, California, recommended an AIDS curriculum for kindergartners, to educate them about the epidemic surrounding them and to allay their fears about the disease. Twenty-two of the twenty-four kindergarten teachers in the district swiftly protested the plan. According to the president of the Palo Alto Board of Education, "Children are not living in a hermetically sealed world." But from the teachers' perspective, "Children are already being robbed of the innocence that should typify youth." The teachers wrote in their letter of protest, "We know that times have changed. Our society has gradually chipped away at the very essence of childhood." Rather than allaying their anxiety, the teachers felt that telling the children about AIDS would simply heighten their fears of the world.[9]

The conflict revolved around the "enlightenment" of children. The school board president harkened back to his own childhood and recalled his anxiety hearing radio reports or conversations about Nazi Germany with no explanations from his parents. He wanted to alleviate this angst for the present generation of children, faced not with the Holocaust but with the contemporary plague of AIDS. The assumption underlying his well-meant intention is that children want to know, have a right to know, and will be soothed by knowing. The teachers, who care for the children each day, did not view their charges as either so savvy or so inquisitive. For them, kindergarten should be preserved as a "children's garden" (its direct translation from German), a time and place sheltered from the trials and tribulations of adult life.

The conflict reflects our split image of childhood: the innocent or the enlightened. On the one hand we have the cherub, an innocent creature cavorting through the woods of childhood, and, on the other, the miniature adult, a highly developed and mature individual in child form. Under pressure to calm the ensuing confusion, we attempt to weld these two images into a third, singular portrait of childhood. We arrive at something akin to the figure of the mythological minotaur—half bull and half man. Only this time we have half adult and half child—the "kinderdult."

It is an ill-fitting union, the cherub and the miniature adult, and this third image, the kinderdult, creates a very odd and unintegrated portrayal of a child. It generates an endless barrage of dilemmas for parents: Is two-year-old Sarah ready for the Tots and Toddlers Preschool or is she too young for institutional care? Is eight-year-old Seth unreasonable in his attempt to veto the parents' decision on next summer's vacation? Can ten-year-old Monica stay home alone after school or should she continue to go to grandmother's? Should fifteen-year-old Pat be allowed to set his own curfew?

It would be far better to replace the kinderdult with a concept that acknowledges that children have many more capabilities than we may have given them credit for in the past, but at the same time progress along lines of development that make them very different than adults and therefore they must constantly be reevaluated as they grow from tiny to little to middle sized to full grown. Until we do that, we are stuck with the absurdity of the kinderdult. This new concept of childhood is yet another reflection of parents' confusion, but it is also a key to breaking the code of perilous parenting and spoiled childhood, as we ask how a mother or father is to raise such a creature, half adult–half child.

UNTANGLING THE KNOTS IN PARENTAL CONFUSION

We are not sociologists when we parent our children. Instead, it is a very personal, psychological experience. What I mean is that we are not thinking about the cuts in educational budgets at 3:30 P.M. when we are at work and get a frantic phone call from our son about his homework assignment due the very next morning. We try to respond to our son's schoolwork meltdown with him over the phone as we push our own work assignments and responsibilities to the side. We do not think about reduced government spending, we just tear our hair out, agonizing that we are not there in person to help, asking ourselves what we have done wrong that our boy cannot grasp the basics of this academic task, and wondering how we are going to get all our own work done before we have to go pick up our younger daughter at day care by 5:15.

But neither are we psychologists when we care for our children. We barely have a moment to take a look inside at our own psychology, emotions, and inner thoughts and fantasies. We are often not even aware of our vacillations between overindulgence and self-involvement. The swings operate at an unconscious level. We have little time for introspection and our struggle just to get through the day often denies us access to the deepest recesses of our own psyches, which contribute to parenting being the peril it is today.

Certainly, if we exercised such introspection all the time our relationships with our children would lose their spontaneity and vitality and become a stilted, overly self-conscious endeavor. Nonetheless, greater insight into our parenting conundrums could help us greatly. We know something is awry, we fear that we are spoiling our sons' and daughters' childhoods, but we are handicapped by a lack of conscious awareness of the roots of confusion that reign over our parenting.

In my clinical work, I hold to the premise that insight is a key to change. This involves making the unconscious conscious and the confusing more explicable. I am inviting readers to share this premise with me and engage in a process of allowing the words in this book to resonate with their own experiences to bring their own confusions in parenting to the light of day. At the same time, just as feminism brought to recognition women's collective experience, I hope, in untangling the knot of parental confusion, to show that one's individual struggle raising a child is also a social phenomenon shared by many and capable of being changed for the better by all of us together.

The reality is that parenting today in America is a deeply personal experience and at the same time a profoundly social experience. To both assess and change the stresses of parenting today, we have to investigate deeply inside our psyches as well as broadly across the landscape of social and economic conditions in this country. This book is about the ways in which social, cultural, and psychological changes have come together with a new definition of a child to create a situation in which parenthood carries the risk of spoiling childhood. Some of that risk is of parents' own making; some is socially imposed.

We need not think of ourselves as either pawns in a larger social game or victims of the larger social order. Conditions exist outside our immediate control that indeed make parenting difficult, such as shrinking opportunities for our children and the increased financial costs of supporting a family. But in as much as we also claim some personal responsibility for confused or harried parenting, we can take charge of shifting our destiny, finding solutions to make parenting sane and childhood healthy.

In fundamental ways, the contemporary plight of parenting is experienced by anyone in charge of raising a child today. At the same time, it will certainly vary by category—age, gender, ethnicity, socioeconomic status. Although we can expect variations, these are the central themes I want to highlight: alarming swings between over- and underparenting because of no time to parent, internal and external pressures to parent well, no supports to do it, and unclear images of both parenthood and childhood. My own narrative is about the middle class, but I believe we will find these strains in other communities of parents as well.

The chapters in this book are aimed at analyzing and finding solutions to the perils of parenting and spoiled childhood. We will look at parents' entrance into parenthood; their dreams and hopes for their children; their specific dilemmas in raising a child who will be successful, self-confident, and loving; and the effects of their ministrations, conflicts, and experiences on the children. We will look at the struggles in raising a kinderdult and the relationship between the kinderdult and the paradox of self-indulgent/overindulgent parenting. We will zero in on two particularly vulnerable aspects of parenting today—our dilemmas about our children's achievement and about our own authority. By the end I hope to have answered the child-rearing riddle with which I started: How can the same generation of parents simultaneously be accused of being the most self-centered, narcissistic set of mothers and fathers in history *and* indulgent, hovering caregivers who fawn over, cater to, and dote on their children in a manner heretofore never seen?

I opened the pages of this book with a quote from Joan Ryan, columnist for the *San Francisco Chronicle,* a parent who would like us all to return to Planet Earth. To that end, she recommends that parents who overanalyze "stop reading articles in Redbook and McCall's with the headlines '10 Ways to Stop Temper Tantrums' and '10 Simple Steps to Better Parenting.' It's silly to think that all advice works for everyone." As an alternative, "maybe we should trust our own instincts. Maybe we don't need a parents' version of The Rules."[10] Unfortunately, our instincts are muddled by our conflicts as we parent today. But I share her skepticism about the usefulness of checklists and ten-step guides. In that spirit, this is not a how-to book; you will not find directives or rules at the end of each chapter. For those of you who have children, I invite you instead to think in new and more conscious ways about your experience as a parent as you read through the pages of *Spoiling Childhood,* and then see where that leads you. The solutions I offer are embedded throughout, in the form of stories and ideas about alternative ways to understand and relate to your children and to yourselves as parents.

I am back in my friend's living room with Miranda on her Big Wheel. I might not have looked so askance at their parenting if Miranda's parents had recognized that it was unreasonable or not in Miranda's best interest to allow her to do what she pleased when she pleased in the name of creative, free expression and adult-like autonomy. They might have been able to intervene more effectively and ask Miranda to stop if they could have seen her as more than a young cherub incapable of being told "No" or being redirected. They might have felt freer to ask that Miranda think about others if they had recognized that Miranda was expressing that she saw herself as the center of the universe but also would welcome someone curbing her self-centeredness. And, ultimately, they might have done better by Miranda if they had also been aware that they were taking the easy way out by avoiding a power struggle with Miranda so as to assuage their own guilt about not being there enough and about occasionally being less than kind, generous, and accepting parents. They would have been able to see more clearly that asking Miranda to do a more quiet activity would be a better option for helping Miranda develop care and concern for others and for moving her out of a very egocentric orbit. They might have provided us all with a quieter meal and eliminated my own older children's question, "Mom, how come they let Miranda do that?"

Just a slice in time with close family friends, but a signifier of the kind of work we each need to do to provide our children with a healthy childhood. To that end, I offer the following chapters, in an attempt to shed light on the external conditions and the personal experiences of child rearing that need to be both understood and changed so as to reduce the perils of parenting today and for generations to come.

CHAPTER TWO

· · · · · ·

Your Majesty, the Baby

*The child shall have a better time than his parents;
he shall not be subject to the necessities which they
have recognized as paramount in life. Illness, death,
renunciation of enjoyment, restriction of his own
will, shall not touch him; the laws of nature and
society shall be abrogated in his favour; he shall
once more really be the centre and core of
creation—"His Majesty the Baby."*
—SIGMUND FREUD[1]

Some years ago I asked a group of thirty-five mothers from a broad range of socioeconomic and ethnic backgrounds to think back to their own childhoods and count how many rooms in their homes held children's clothes, toys, artwork, or paraphernalia. The overwhelming response from this group of women, ranging in age from twenty-five to forty-five, was "One." Then I asked them to think of their own homes today. How many of the rooms contained either their children's clothes, toys, possessions, or artistic creations? A self-conscious giggle rippled through the group as they responded in unison, "Just about every room in the house." One woman even admitted to adding a shed to her house to handle the spillover of her son's toys.

This is not just an example of the increased material indulgence of parents today. As the child moves from a single room to fill every corner of the house, we witness the tremendous importance and centrality placed on this generation of children. We might even say we actually *overvalue* our children. Allowing them to take up so much space in contrast to our own parents' ways is simply a reflection of this overvaluation, an overvaluation that marks our generation and is a prime contributor to the peril of parenting.

If you call Leslie's house, you will hear four-year-old Magda's voice on the answering machine. With Leslie's prompting, her daughter, Magda, greets you, sings a song, falters for several seconds, and then says, "Good-bye." For the caller, it seems to take a very long time. Two years ago, Magda's parents separated. Before Magda's birth, her parents had a loving and passionate relationship. Since her birth, Magda had been allowed to take up every corner of psychological space in her parents' lives. Any small sign of distress was taken very seriously by mother. Therefore, Magda slept with her mother every night. Her father, Matthew, was relegated to another bed. An only child, Magda was never left out of her parents' sight. Because the parents were work partners in an accounting firm, Magda accompanied them to work every day for her first two years. Her needs took precedence over work obligations at all times. Ultimately, the marriage fell apart, as there was no room for the couple to have a life outside of catering to Magda's needs. The clinician who assessed three-year-old Magda and her family in a postdivorce evaluation concluded that both Leslie and Matthew were very caring and devoted parents to a well-loved, ebullient child, but they had raised Magda to the level of a deity, and she was at risk for being stuck at a two-year-old level in which she would always expect the world to revolve around her.

Do we want to relegate our children back to one room in the house or put our own needs over theirs in early life? No, but we would do well to check our tendencies to let our children, their possessions, and their psyches take full reign of both our homes and our existences. Leslie and Matthew's marriage might have been saved and Magda might not have been placed in a high-risk category if someone could have stepped in earlier to help Leslie and Matthew do exactly that. Not just Leslie and Matthew, but all of us need help checking our tendencies to overvalue our children. We can begin by getting insight into *why* we have come to overvalue our children, *how* we overvalue them, and *why* it is important to change that.

Today's parents are definitely perceived as seeing their children as very, very special, maybe even like royalty. To coin a phrase from Sigmund Freud, it is typical for all new mothers and fathers to see our little charges as "your majesty, the baby."[2] With a second chance to make up for all the ways our own parents did not raise us well and with this new little person who comes from us and will represent us in the world, we all engage in soaring fantasies about who our children will be and what they will accomplish in their lives.

But middle-class parents today may have gone overboard in such fantasies about their children. Books with titles such as "The Too Precious Child[3] suggest that professionals, at least, are worried about this. They alert us to the possibility that we may have a new, majestic child, whose presence fills every corner of the house and who is more special and "royal" than Freud could ever have imagined some eighty years ago when he first made reference to "your majesty, the baby." The concern is not just that parents overvalue their children, but that they do this because they themselves are very narcissistic. Caught up in their own grandiosity and self-centeredness, they extend this to their children by overglorifying and perceiving the same grandeur in the children as well.

Something has gone awry in the fantasies about and attitudes toward our children. Our reveries have become overblown and, at the same time, laced with anxieties. Recognizing that we are a generation whose soaring fantasies have spiraled out of control will put us in much better stead for controlling our propensity to go overboard in raising our children to the level of deities. How do we mend it so we don't continue to overvalue our children in ways that are not healthy for them? This is the question I would like to address now in turning to a discussion of "your majesty, the baby."

YOUR COMMODITY, THE BABY

First we need to look more closely at parents' actual attitudes toward their little ones. Besides letting children fill up every corner of the house, what evidence do we have that parents today overvalue their children?

Once a baby comes into the world, some middle-class parents use their babies to broadcast their own status in the world, to be their showpieces. In the 1980s, we heard media reports exposing parents' lavish indulgence of their children. *Business Week* reported on a twenty-seven-year-old mother who bought her eight-month-old son twenty-five jogging suits, a tuxedo, and a ninety-dollar corduroy suit, confiding, "Let's face it, my kid is an extension of myself, and I have a good time dressing him up."[4] This mother represents the extreme and by the 1990s, with the economy taking a downturn and people tightening their financial belts, we hear less of such extravagances, but the commentary on the American middle-class parent holds firm: Today's mothers and fathers indulge their children, heap unnecessary extravagances upon them, and lack common sense when it comes to their narcissistic investment in their children. A baby has so much "stimulation" paraphernalia in his crib that you cannot find him amidst the toys. A one-year-old shows up to her first birthday party in an eighty-dollar Laura Ashley dress. Even people without financial resources will blow a large chunk of their income on items for the children. What meaning does a child have to parents that would drive them to such extravagances?

To answer this question we must first put the entrance into parenthood in social context. Many middle-class parents today were several years into adulthood before they had children. Some waited so as to get their careers in order first or to extend their years of liberation, a defining characteristic of the Peter Pan generation, which never wanted to grow up. Some thought they did not want children at all, seeing parenthood as interfering with other ambitions. Only later, as they entered their thirties or forties, did the desire to parent surface, when either the biological or the existential clock began to tick very loudly. If parenthood is, at least in part, a means of ensuring one's immortality, there is nothing like a midlife crisis to jolt a person into the realization that he or she might actually die or become infertile before getting a chance to procreate and therefore live forever.

People becoming parents for the first time in their thirties are largely responsible for the 3.7 million births in the United States recorded in 1985, the highest number in twenty years.[5] The number of women thirty-five or over who were giving birth for the first time quadrupled from the late 1970s to the late 1980s.[6] Whereas some people postponed parenthood, others were unable to find acceptable partners with whom to parent. And still others, skeptical about the viability of a partnership at all in an age of rampant relationship failures, grappled with the practical, emotional, and, for some, moral issues of parenting without a partner.

In past generations, having a child was simply what one did soon after marriage. Anything else was considered a serious aberration, a problem in the marriage, or a pitiable state of infertility. Today, this is no longer true. With increased choices, the actual decision about becoming a parent is very weighty, perhaps almost fetishized. In 1989, an ad for a seminar sponsored by Children's Hospital of San Francisco appeared in the *San Francisco Examiner*. Entitled "Baby Talk," it was not about where to buy diapers or what to do if your baby has colic. Instead, the morning half of the program was billed as, "Pregnancy and Parenthood after 35." The ad told a perspective attendee, "You're over 35 and considering kids. It's a big decision. You must consider the emotional investment, the dramatic changes to your life-style and any medical risks."[7]

It is admirable to ask people to give careful thought to the actualities of raising a child, for this is a lifetime commitment that cannot be undone. But the ante is raised when we highlight and organize paid programs around the tremendous investment, dramatic change, and risk, rather than approaching the transition to parenting as part of the natural, unfolding developmental progression of adulthood. We all know that becoming a parent is a shock, one we can know only by going through it. The fetishism comes when this aspect of parenting is underscored, commodified, and taught to a group of people who are already ripe for overvaluation or glorification of any investment they make.

In the new context of "big decision" for parents, it is not surprising that "Baby," at least in concept, looms bigger than life, as the entity that will both govern and potentially make or break one's future. This attitude toward the baby affects not only the older parent who has waited a long time to have a child, but permeates the consciousness of adults of all ages. Once you have answered the big decision in the affirmative, you have to believe that the trouble will be worth it and that the prize will be grand.

Sylvia is a mother-to-be of thirty-three. Each morning she awakens and has a little talk with her fetus. She has eight different books by her bedside about raising a happy and healthy child. Her husband, Larry, has had the sonogram slides of their baby blown up into poster size and has already sent copies of the sonogram videotape to grandparents, aunts, and uncles. Four different baby showers are in the making. Sylvia and Larry's celebration of their child is reinforced by the culture surrounding them, where we now find that infants and small children have their own special stores, perfumes, nursery gadgets, and parent training manuals to guide their mothers and fathers in how to raise them.

Ironically, although the American birth rate exploded in the latter years of the 1980s, there is a simultaneous sense of babies as a scarce commodity. In the afternoon of the "Baby Talk" seminar referred to above, one could now become educated about infertility: "You want children but are having trouble conceiving." The postponement of parenthood until a later age, increased and extended use of mechanical and chemical forms of birth control, and carelessly monitored but frightening environmental intrusions, such as chronic low-dose radiation, have left growing numbers of women and men infertile. Some couples have to go through several medical or surgical interventions and several years before a child is conceived. Others who have not yet even attempted pregnancy imagine that such might also be their fate. For many, fertility efforts fail, leaving people with no chance of their own biological child.

Even with the advent of artificial insemination, *in vitro* fertilization, egg donorship, and surrogate motherhood, as well as the age-old institution of adoption, parents-to-be are not encouraged that a baby is within their reach. The number of domestic babies available for adoption has decreased, as a result of legalized abortion, better access to effective birth control, and greater acceptance of single women keeping their babies. And the costs of alternative birth technologies are exorbitant, the time and medical and emotional involvement long and intense, and the success rates fairly low.

Accompanying the sense of babies being scarce is the feeling that is even more central to modern parenthood: Things that are thought to be hard to come by become more valuable, and so it is that babies today can come to be seen as very *precious*. Precious babies can be bought by renting out another woman's womb or purchased through pouring tens of thousands of dollars into private adoption searches. Precious babies are sometimes acquired in exchange for years of physical pain, psychological anguish, and depleted bankbooks on the consumer's part. Precious babies are looked upon enviously by those who do not come by one easily when one is in the arms of someone who did. Whether done the "old-fashioned" way or through adoption or newfangled technology, having a child is now felt to be a remarkable phenomenon done against great odds.

Before an infant has even entered the world and had the opportunity to become the object of the parents' fantasies of unbridled opportunities and limitless freedoms, it has been assigned royalty status. It takes no more than the mother and father's belief in the rarity of their little baby's conception to usher in the coronation. And the ascendance to the throne is ensured by the imagined enormity of the infant's impact on the lives of those in the kingdom waiting to serve it.

Is it any wonder, then, that the stage is set, upon arrival, for the baby to be treated as precious cargo forever after? Sylvia and Larry's celebrated fetus becomes the child whose artwork covers every wall in the house and whose every move is greeted with admiration. This child has a hard time recognizing that her needs will not always come first and that every small act will not be accompanied by bells and whistles. Had Sylvia and Larry been counseled before the birth of their child that "natural" childbirth is best accompanied by an excited but low-key attitude toward their baby, and had they been warned that their inflated celebration might create an omnipotent child intent on ruling the world, they might have turned their attention to curbing their overvaluation. But this would be best accomplished if they could also bring to consciousness the psychological forces that have led them to such overvaluation in the first place. The child as precious commodity is only one factor pushing parents toward overvaluation. Let us now turn to the others.

IF IT'S NOT PERFECT, "BREAK IT"

As the child-to-be becomes precious, it is predictable that when one actually comes along, the parents are going to want a perfect one. This desire is fueled by a scientific community that has discovered that one can actually tamper with Mother Nature in striving toward perfection.

New birth technologies can screen for genetic anomalies, tell the sex of an unborn child, and correct malformations and potentially fatal abnormalities before a baby leaves the womb. These scientific advances infuse us with a belief that we will have greater and greater control over our new child's destiny. No longer does the dictum hold, "You take what is given to you and make the best of it." Instead, with access to increased technological knowledge, we can choose to terminate the impending birth of a seriously malformed or abnormal fetus or attempt to fix one that shows up less than perfect. As a six-year-old little friend of mine told his father about the approaching amniocentesis of his pregnant mother, "I get it. If the baby's not right, we'll take it out and break it."

Whether science informs psyche or psyche dictates the direction of science or a reciprocal feedback loop exists between the two, the following reality holds. Mothers and fathers and even their children are deeply affected by the technological transformation of baby making and birth from natural phenomena to medical procedures that strive for perfection. So we begin to accept the idea that, "If the baby's not right, fix it or take it out and break it."

This new consciousness allows perspective parents to terminate a pregnancy that might otherwise culminate in a tragic birth with lifelong consequences for both child and family. It supports the rights of women and men to take control over their own lives and make informed decisions about the lives they may be bringing into the world. It allows us to enter the womb and make alterations in the baby before it has even met the world.

But as is often true in such delicate matters, the new consciousness that has developed—"breaking it" if it's not right or if we can't fix it—simultaneously reveals a darker side of our sensibilities regarding the striving for perfection. Occasionally we hear newsworthy stories about incidents of parents who relinquish their disabled or adopted children because of the tremendous difficulties in raising the children.[8] As a mental health professional, I also see the phenomenon in the consulting room. Recently I completed a consultation with a colleague who was working with a family on the verge of giving their ten-year-old niece up for adoption. They had taken her in with the plan of adopting her themselves. But she just wasn't working out as well as they would have wished. She was a behavior problem and fairly sullen much of the time. She wasn't performing very well at school. She had not bonded with her new parents in the way they had hoped. The therapy had not "fixed" the girl as they had anticipated. The reality did not match the soaring fantasies they had of repair, transformation, and glory when they had taken this girl in two years earlier. My colleague did not feel confident that she could turn the tides on their wish to relinquish the girl. This would have required reexamining their fantasies and motivation for becoming parents to their niece. It would have meant exploring in more depth the meaning of her seemingly recalcitrant symptoms, to understand them as a communication of her distress, a protest against all that happened to her before, and a test of the resiliency of her new parents. It would have entailed inviting the couple to develop a more realistic sense of what they might expect from this child and their relationship with her. It would have required relinquishing their fantasy of transforming this child. They were not open to such work.

Although it seems counterintuitive, such stories of rejection ("If you're not right, I'll discard you") actually highlight the perception of child as royalty these days. While the overwhelming majority of parents carry their fetuses to term and accept the child who is delivered to them, whether through birth or adoption, we occasionally hear stories of parents who don't. The rare occurrences of relinquishment of less-than-perfect children underscore the deep internalization in our culture of "your majesty, the baby" as the organizing feature in our perception of infanthood and childhood: "If it is not perfect, of majestic proportions, then I do not want it."

Child abandonment, relinquishment, and even infanticide have existed throughout human history, in far worse proportions than we have ever seen in this country. But what is unique to our society now is the obsessive overvaluation that underlies our attitude about both wanted and unwanted children. We are awash in the desire for perfection that stems from overvaluation. Precious babies earn their title as precious by being flawless. This can be understood as an anxious defense against the worry that, if it is not perfect, it will not be lovable and, more importantly, *I* will not be able to love it. Maybe I won't even want it.

Psychologist Miriam Elson refers to the emotional blow incurred when a child *is* born with congenital defects. It is a profound narcissistic trauma for parents, accompanied by a deep loss of self-esteem.[9] With the advent of medical technology and fine scrutiny of the child's well-being through machines and tests, the possibility of this kind of trauma or disappointment is heightened, for we now learn much more about our child's imperfections and more infants with deficits are kept alive through advanced technology. The angst that one's baby is at risk for defect can occur as early as the embryo stage when the child-to-be fails to appear as a perfect fetal image on the sonogram screen. With the widespread use of amniocentesis and other new forms of fetal screening, it has become a normal developmental stage of expectant parenthood to go through a month or so of worry and "what ifs" until receiving test results about the health of the baby.

Relatedly, the new ideology of the birth technologies—that many maladies can either be fixed or avoided—further eats away at middle-class parents. It pressures them into feeling that baby perfection is within their reach. It eliminates the idea that buffered past generations and still does for poorer people today—because there is nothing one can do to prevent it, one just has to accept what one gets, which might well be an unhealthy baby or one who may never live to adulthood. Without that buffer and with the expectation of a child who will absolutely outlive the parents, we find that in the parent's psyche, the quest for perfection is constantly shadowed by the fear of catastrophe.

If parenthood is a time for men and women to herald a rebirth of feelings of endless possibility and limitless horizons, the specter of birth defect and developmental disaster undermines the natural unfolding of soaring fantasies on the part of mothers and fathers today. Esther and Barry marvel in their new little daughter, Myrna—her round, angelic face; her quick responsiveness; her sweet disposition. But the fetal heart monitor strapped to Esther during her labor announced several minutes of fetal distress for Myrna before the doctor ordered a cesarean section. Newborn Myrna showed glowing reports on her Apgar scores, except that she was a little low on oxygen. In the back of Esther and Barry's minds is the gnawing worry that birth trauma may lead to learning disabilities down the line. To keep their fears at bay, they pump up the volume on their dreams for their child, drowning out the voice of doom. A classic situation where an ounce of knowledge culminates in a ton of pain, "enlightened" birth propels the parents into overvaluation and genuflection toward their miracle majesties because they know all too well the potential for other than a majesty.

This type of overvaluation of the child is a psychological defense on the parents' part. It is an attempt on the parents' part to resolve their agonizing inner tension between perfection and catastrophe. If they can only believe that their child is precious and perfect, they can ward off the morbid fear that their opportunity for soaring fantasies will be rudely torn from them through developmental disaster.

Medical technology and modern psychology only serve to heighten the need for this defense. Parents are alerted to all that can go wrong for their child while at the same time being primed always to expect that perfection is within their reach. Medical technology inflates the notion that parents can hold reign over nature. Psychology picks up the ball in promoting the notion of personal growth and improvement through our own efforts. Burdened with the feeling that, if something *does* go wrong, parents can and should fix it, parents inflate the image of "your majesty, the baby" even more, as a psychological insurance policy against developmental disaster.

The inflated "your majesty, the baby" as a defense against the conflict between perfection and disaster extends well beyond the experience of parents of newborns. It afflicts us throughout our child-rearing years, as we come to realize that not just developmental disaster but an unfriendly world threatens our children's well-being. Our own First Lady and child advocate, Hillary Rodham Clinton, reminds us: "Everywhere we look, children are under assault: from violence and neglect, from the breakup of families, from the temptations of alcohol, tobacco, sex, and drug abuse, from greed, materialism, and spiritual emptiness. These problems are not new, but in our time they have skyrocketed."[10] The fact that the future, and even the present, does not look so sanguine for our children puts a real dent in our soaring dreams for them.

Tiffany is a mother who comes from a long line of musicians. She herself is one, leaving her middle class but penny poor. Her daughter, Tamika, also shows wonderful musical talent and enjoys playing her instruments. Tiffany has dreams of her daughter getting a scholarship to Julliard. She wants Tamika's musical future to be less of a struggle than hers was—she had to work two jobs and swap housecleaning for violin lessons all the way through high school. She has fought successfully to enroll her child in a public school outside of her district because of their superb musical program. She has no money to provide her child private lessons. Last week she received a school notice announcing the permanent closure of their music program, due to budget shortages. She opened the paper this week only to learn about drastic cuts in federal funding for the arts. She is in tears. How will her dreams for her daughter ever come true?

As we feel thwarted in our strong "second chance" desire to give our children a better life than the one we once had, we feel terribly guilty. We feel guilty for not having the omnipotence to make it any better for our children. We feel guilty for being part of the collective entity that made it so bad in the first place. We feel guilty for having it better than our children.

As life goes on, the dreams for our children continue to be bruised by intrusive thoughts and feelings of failure, danger, and limitation. Rather than "your majesty, the baby," we peer down on a son or daughter who to us means *so* much, in a society where a child means so little. Our guilt mounts.

We try to compensate for the guilt, for the disquieting thoughts, by overvaluing our children even more. We firmly center ourselves around our child in the context of a world where we see children pushed to the periphery. The precious and perfect child will assure us that the world won't be as bad to our children as we fear.

This is exactly how Tiffany handled her dreams for her daughter in the face of a budgetary system where music no longer counted for very much. Rather than giving up on her reveries about Tamika's future, she expounded on the fantasies even more. In her eyes, Tamika was elevated from a talented little musician to a musical genius. Tiffany devoted the next several months to practicing both violin and piano with Tamika many hours a day, despite Tamika's protests that this was really a little too intense for her. She spent hour after hour on the Internet exploring every available program or scholarship for musically gifted children. Each morning she woke up and reminded Tamika of what a future she had as a virtuoso. And each night she went to bed anxious that her daughter's musical future was being rudely torn from her.

So glorifying "your majesty, the baby" extends from birth to maturity. Already intoxicated by the concept of having a child well before the child leaves the womb, the too precious neonate soon becomes the too precious child, facing a world with an overabundance of both parental involvement and hand wringing. Mothers and fathers dream of themselves as perfect parents to the perfect child, but a nightmare lurks beneath.

Middle-class parents no longer have to worry whether their child will physically survive; instead, what they want for their child is a happy and fulfilling future, to think that their child is special, and to let the child know so.[11] Yet underlying the quest for happiness is the gnawing fear that such happiness, and even physical survival, is not guaranteed. Even middle-class children die—from sudden infant death syndrome, from cancer and incurable disease, from accidents, from violence, from suicide. And plenty of children are unhappy. Yet parents are told that *they* are the ones ultimately responsible for their child's future. Without the requisite time or supporting social structures to secure that future for their children, parents are left riddled with anxiety. As if having discovered they've been sold the Brooklyn Bridge, parents experience a sensation, either conscious or unconscious, and tinged with anxiety, that "this isn't the way it was supposed to be." Raising the children to the level of deities is an unconscious attempt to drown out this troubling thought.

NARCISSISM

We must return to another component of parents' overvaluation of their children: parents' narcissism. It would seem that this is what makes parents ripe for worrying about their children's every little imperfection, overglorifying the children's every move, and being disappointed with anything short of a flawless child.

However, although I do think that this generation's sense of self-involvement and grandiosity plays its part in the overvaluation of the children, the relationship between parents' narcissism and "your majesty, the baby" is extremely complex. To begin, let us be clear about what we are referring to when we talk about parents' narcissism.

When we ourselves were first born, we experienced ourselves as the center of the universe and expected others to revolve around us. This is known as "primary narcissism." As we grew, we shed that early narcissistic state and learned about give and take with others. We developed a relationship with the world that became informed by our capacity for care and concern for those around us.

Upon becoming parents, we are given a little freedom to become narcissistic once again, with no aspersion cast on our character. Sigmund Freud, talking about "your majesty, the baby," put it this way: "If we look at the attitude of affection in parents toward their children, we have to recognize that it is a revival and reproduction of their own narcissism, which they have long since abandoned."[12] This narcissism takes the form of our soaring fantasies about our offspring. I would dub this "expectable parental narcissism." It is a reactivation of that early state when the world revolved around us and we felt that nothing but us counted, only now those feelings are focused on the new baby rather than on ourselves. This reactivation of our early narcissistic state is what accounts for the overvaluation of our child.

Expectable parental narcissism is the mother gazing lovingly at her four-month-old son with hope and joy in her eyes as she confidently cradles him in her arms. It is the father dreaming of a life of success and happiness for his daughter as he shields her from loud noises in the next room.

We are given full license to fantasize for our child a limitless potential, as long we do not completely lose our grip on reality. We can reexperience our own early narcissism, as long as we are simultaneously capable of focusing on the infant as a separate person in need of care and attention and as long we also don't forget to help our child develop those very capacities for care and concern that will someday allow him or her to become a good parent.

In other words, a certain degree of narcissism is actually a positive thing in parenting. It is perfectly normal and to be found among all good parents. But today's parents are accused of being overly narcissistic, never relinquishing the early state of narcissism when they were absorbed only with themselves. Are parents overstepping the boundaries of *expectable* parental narcissism as they receive the late twentieth-century majesties, the babies, into their lives?

In previous generations there have been parents who were accused of fulfilling their own needs for aggrandizement by having their children achieve for them. But now an entire generation of parents, not just a pathological few, is called narcissistic. So preoccupied with their own needs, they simply absorb the children into their adult lives, rather than carving out space around the children. The children must be glorified to satisfy the parents' hunger for glory. This earns the parents the pejorative label of "narcissist."

No doubt there are parents today who are so blind to their children as separate people and so focused on their own desires and needs that parenting becomes an act of obliteration rather than nurturance. They overvalue their children only in the same way that they overvalue themselves and just to show how wonderful they themselves are.

Frederick and Jocelyn come to me for a parenting consultation. They are both very accomplished professionals. They have brought a thick portfolio of their child's most recent accomplishments, along with several photographs of her to demonstrate her beauty. Kristen is only four. They want her to have every opportunity for success, and they believe that when she grows up she will be a concert pianist like her grandfather. They marvel at what a shining star they have produced, and are elated that they have the ability to provide her with all the things they never had. There's only one little problem. Kristen falls apart every time she has to go to her music lesson. Can I help her get over that?

When Frederick and Jocelyn could see that their daughter's tantrums were a cry for help rather than a symptom that needed to be eliminated, they began to take stock of their overinvestment and self-centered wants for their child. I asked them each to spend some time observing and reflecting on who Kristen actually was and then tell their thoughts to each other. They were not to focus on the things Kristen could do, but more on what she liked and didn't like, what her daily rhythms were like, what things made her happy or distressed, and what her personality was like. The therapeutic goal was to acknowledge Kristen as a little girl, not a deity. This was extremely hard for them, as their observations were initially blurred by their own grandiose fantasies of who Kristen should be. But with time they were able to lift the veil of their own visions for their child and step back and see that Kristen really just wanted to be left alone in her own fantasy world where she could play out her own imaginary dramas with little figures. Rather than stopping the tantrums, they stopped the music lessons, and the tantrums took care of themselves. Working both with each other and with a third party (myself), their efforts paid off in helping them develop greater sensitivity to their child as just a little person, albeit special, with her own needs and wants. There would be plenty of time later for music lessons, when (or if) Kristen expressed *her* desire to take classes.

But most parents that I meet are not like Frederick and Jocelyn. They do not fit the simple profile of narcissistic parents who aggrandize their child for their own glory. They present a much more complicated picture. Don and Gloria have dreams that their five-year-old little son will some day be a star tennis player like his father, but they worry that his forceps delivery may have damaged the part of his brain needed for the fast pace and hand–eye coordination of tennis. They imagine that he might end up a trial lawyer like his grandfather, given his love of words and public speaking—with the coffee table as his podium. But they're discouraged that this will ever happen, when neither of them is home enough to engage in the kind of conversation that would further develop his forensic skills. Don and Gloria's soaring dreams, laced with worry, are more typically what I see in my consulting room.

Without intervention, Don and Gloria's little boy, Daniel, could have been headed for trouble. His parents came to me because Daniel was having difficulty sleeping at night and was demanding that his parents help him with every little thing he did, wanting to do it perfectly but never feeling confident that he could get there on his own. He grew frustrated easily and gave up when things got a little hard. He had picked up on the tension between his parents' dreams and worries and had begun to internalize them as his own. He was headed for an anxiety disorder.

Like with Kristen, I decided it was more important to work with Daniel's parents than to bring Daniel into my office. But, Don and Gloria were harder nuts to crack than Frederick and Jocelyn. Their high hopes and worries were all tangled up with each other and ran deep into their psyches. I diagnosed them as suffering from what I call the "wounding of expectable parental narcissism." It is a diagnosis particular to our generation. Growing up expecting to have it all, we are ripe for dreaming about our children as great tennis players, lawyers, and so on, and wringing our hands at the thought that it could come to any less than that. But then our dreams collapse when they are intruded on by fantasies of impending disaster—in Don and Gloria's case because of damage through the birth canal or understimulation through parental absence. The double-edged blade of medical progress that promises transcendence but forebodes disaster, combined with an era of worries about an uncertain future, crashed head on with Don and Gloria's fantasies. At an unconscious level, they then experienced a piercing of the parental narcissism that was to be their birthright in having a child.

The only way I could work with Don and Gloria was to bring this tension between dream and disaster to consciousness. Unlike Frederick and Jocelyn, who were unbridled in their narcissistic behavior toward their child, Don and Gloria had not felt free to be "narcissistic" enough, in the sense of entertaining unencumbered soaring fantasies for their little boy. Their fantasies kept getting bruised by imagined calamities.

My first job was to address their guilt head on. In their first session, they focused solely on all the ways they had either damaged their son or left him unprotected from bad things that could befall him. I asked them to consider instead the good things they were providing for their son. This was an eye-opener for them. Astonishingly, they had never given it much thought. I also asked them to pay attention to all the ways they might be communicating their worries to their son. This took several weeks, but over time they came to recognize that the flip side of Daniel always demanding help was them hovering over him with bated breath wondering whether he really was going to be able to complete successfully the tasks he had started. They began to give him some breathing space.

Only then did I introduce the next piece of work, which was similar to what I had zeroed in on immediately with Frederick and Jocelyn. What were their dreams for Daniel, where did they come from, and would it be so terrible if Daniel fell short of them? Perhaps they were too caught up in overvaluing his every move, in trying to assure both him and themselves of Daniel's perfection and of his escape from disaster. At this point, they grew angry with me and defended themselves, saying they were just trying to give Daniel a good start and foster his self-esteem. But when I asked them if it was working, they grew quiet and reconsidered what they were doing. We began to look at their lethal combination of wonderment and worry. As they relaxed both their worries and their overblown fantasies about Daniel, they encouraged him to do things on his own and stressed that having fun doing something was more important than doing it perfectly. Over time, Daniel was released from being the repository of Gloria and Don's intermingled hopes and horrors. His own anxiety symptoms subsided and he was better able to sleep through the night.

Without insight or intervention, parents like Don and Gloria can get caught in a web of contradictory forces that only reinforces the wounding of their expectable parental narcissism and sometimes makes it look like *pathological* narcissism. On one side of the web is the present structure of work in America, which does not make it easy for parents to "decenter" around their children—that is, to place their children, rather than themselves, at the focal point of attention. To highlight this, let me tell you the story of a colleague of mine. Although ultimately reversing their first decision, the American Board of Child and Family Psychiatry initially turned down her psychiatry residency as insufficient training because she had not fulfilled the standard requirement of the usual two-year full-time residency. Instead, she had arranged an extension of her residency to four years, working half-time to allow ample time to devote to her two young children. Consider the irony of the initial denial of her work/parenting plan by an organization that purports to foster the psychological well-being of children and families. It was not my colleague but her work environment that demanded that she be more narcissistic, punishing her for attempting to attend to her children rather than focusing solely on her career. The social demand is that she concentrate on herself, not her children.

On the other side of the web are the pressures from *within* us. First is the parents' own sense of entitlement and, indeed, narcissistic tendencies. We are talking about a generation that is not too keen on the idea of growing up and was spoon-fed on the belief, which became deeply internalized, that the world was their oyster. This left

stomach and tears streaming down my face, quietly sobbing, between contractions, "Mine will never come out." But after a while I was able to relax in the belief that I too would have one of those healthy babies soon.

I have always felt deeply indebted to that midwife. I apply what I learned from her to my work with parents' internalized social angst. I try to facilitate a process in which parents can rid themselves of the nightmare of impending doom. If I can help them stop their psychological hyperventilating, like the midwife helped me with my physical breathing, they may be able to awaken themselves to the reality that their child has plenty of opportunities to have success and happiness. I push them to consider that many of their worries are not well founded, but are anxious preoccupations with things that could, but most likely will never happen. Most children are resilient and weather the ups and down of childhood intact. Even in a society that is not kind to children, children from the middle class can most likely count on a roof over their head, a completed education, and a fair amount of choice in both career and personal life. It is better to focus on problems that actually are there, rather than ones of our own imagination. The therapeutic goal is to free ourselves both from the nightmares and from the need to overvalue our child as an insurance policy against disaster.

A friend calls me at least once a month worried sick about the calamities confronting one or the other of her two daughters, whom she sees as very gifted. Each time she is reduced to tears, truly believing that her children's future is close to ruin because of a mediocre teacher, a slight learning problem, a failure of one of her daughters to make friends as easily as my friend would hope for her. She keeps imagining that life would have been better if she had indeed decided to place her daughters in the school for gifted children that would have required two hours of commute time a day. Each time I have to talk her down, first by acknowledging how upset she is, then by offering some solutions to the immediate problem, and only then suggesting that, in the long run, I think this daughter or the other will come out of this "crisis" intact and healthy. But if truth be told, I do hold back in all that I am thinking, because I am being friend, not therapist, and I experience her as staunchly defended against the message I would truly like to deliver: "Look, your kids really don't have it so bad. They have so much going for them, compared to some of the disasters I see in my office each week, so stop wringing your hands and relax and enjoy them." What I would wish for both her and her daughters is that they could rejoice in what is going well and put to rest all the fears of what isn't.

Lightening up or getting a grip is only a first step. After that comes finding an internal brake system on overvaluation. One method to establish such a system is the process I used in enabling Jocelyn and Frederick to let go of their music mania for Kristen—asking the parents to focus on who the child really was, her likes, dislikes, and so forth, rather than concentrating on who they wanted her to be. Another such method can be seen in the case of Don and Gloria, who finally gave Daniel some breathing space and accepted that enjoying doing something cockeyed is better than doing something anxiously to perfection.

I would invite each of us to think about whether we are overvaluing our children to no good end. I would ask us to step outside ourselves and look at the ways in which we may be doing that. Stanley never spoke about his four-year-old son in anything but hyperbole. Little Aaron was an *incredible* skier, had a *phenomenal* ear for music, and was a *genius* with puzzles. We put Stanley's descriptions of his son on audiotape. I then asked Stanley to listen to his own words and to imagine that he was Aaron and what Aaron might feel listening to Stanley's descriptions of him. Would he like it if someone always talked about him that way, particularly someone with whom he was intimately involved? Just listening to his narrative and putting himself in his son's shoes was a wake-up call to Stanley about the kind of pressure he was putting on his little boy in his overblown assessments of him. He discovered that caring did not equate with overvaluing, and that his overvaluation actually was a form of negligence in which he failed to attend to Aaron's real little self and real needs. If he had kept going with his overblown assessments, he would just be playing out his own narcissistic needs and internalized worries, rather than helping Aaron grow into a sturdy, self-confident little boy comfortable with what he *could* do rather than what everyone thought he could (or should) do. Aaron's anxieties about measuring up and performing for other people's pleasures could have left Aaron with either a "false" personality or an overblown sense of himself in which he would internalize all his father's exaggerated descriptions of him as true.

Sometimes I ask parents to imagine adding the word "your majesty" to past interactions with their child. If the label fits, it's a signal of being involved in overvaluation. Then comes the harder step: developing a self-conscious attitude in which we admonish ourselves to "stop it" when we feel the internal pressure to elevate our children to royalty status. Often it simply takes the realization of how we are damaging our children, either by fostering self-centeredness or creating anxiety, to get our overvaluation under control. Other times, it demands a form of consciousness raising where two parents work together to watch for signs in both the other person and themselves that they are engaged in the nasty dance between dreams and disaster that results in overblowing a child's every move and accomplishment.

Curbing our runaway hopes and dreams for our children by fusing them with a more realistic assessment of who our children are, what they really need, and what they actually want can be invaluable in moving us back toward expectable parental narcissism, where hopes and dreams are checked by the realistic boundaries around our child. Establishing internal controls, which will stop us from being carried away in our glorification of our children, can also protect us and our children from our own narcissistic tendencies, where overvaluation of our child is done solely for our own aggrandizement and at the expense of recognizing our child as a separate person. Implementing a brake system might also stop us from allowing the whole house to be taken over by baby's bounty, which I propose will be healthier for parents and children alike.

And so we have the story of "your majesty, the baby." Parents struggle to create a balance of encircling their children with soaring dreams and hopes while at the same time sheltering, protecting, and preparing them for the a world that is perceived as either unfriendly or fraught with danger. They are at risk for overvaluing their child, but, with a greater consciousness of both their own sense of entitlement and unbridled expectations and their unfounded overwrought worries, parents can begin to approach their sons and daughters as healthy, growing children rather than worshipped deities.

CHAPTER THREE

· · · · · ·

And Baby Makes Three, or Is Baby Me?

Good enough parents endeavor to evaluate and respond to matters both from their adult perspective and from the quite different one of the child, and to base their actions on a reasonable integration of the two, while accepting that the child, because of his immaturity, can understand matters only from his point of view.
—BRUNO BETTELHEIM[1]

Parents are stricken by a wounding of expectable parental narcissism. For all of their child-rearing years, in their desire to be even better than good enough parents, they work valiantly to suture that wound. This struggle takes a very particular form: trying to balance a life that is healthy for both parent and child. Today's generation of parents, I believe, is having an especially hard time trying to sort out their own needs from their baby's. They vacillate wildly between catering to their children as the center of the universe and seeing their sons and daughters only through the lens of their own needs.

To be good parents, we need to have developed, early in our own lives a clearly demarcated sense of where we stop and another starts. This capacity goes hand in hand with the relinquishment of one's own earliest solipsistic state of "me, me, me." Unfortunately, both external and internal contemporary forces mitigate against parents' ability to establish clear boundaries between themselves and their children, creating yet another peril of parenting.

It used to be that parenthood was the ultimate marker of adulthood. That is no longer so. The road to adulthood can now be reached through many paths, not just in accordance with the old model of the married couple, two children, and a car. In fact, parenthood today is sometimes seen as an impediment to adult growth and development, as when it interferes with career commitment and advancement. Ask any mother who is trying to balance both.

"First comes love, then comes marriage, then comes Susie with a baby carriage" no longer rings universally true, and most parents pushing baby carriages are also collecting pay checks. Thus, the new, "chosen" child who comes on the scene has very different meaning to the parent than the inevitable infant of yesteryear. When baby arrives, parents today have a tremendously difficult time attending to both their own adult needs and those of their child. The problem runs much deeper than the juggling act of balancing career and family. Psychologically, mothers and fathers, each in their own way, continually grapple with recognizing the line that signals where they stop and their children start.

Moira tells me that the only way she can get respite from parenting is to go far away from her children for awhile, even across the continent. When she's with them, which is usually after intensive hours of work as an academic at a local college, she finds herself close to tears any time one of them cries. Their pain is hers. She worries about them incessantly. She assumes they are worried, too. When one did not get into the school of his choice, she imagined he was devastated. He didn't seem to care so much. Hovering over them in their presence, she then flees as the only way she knows to establish psychological boundaries between herself and her children.

Joel, a financial advisor, is a divorced father of an eight-year-old boy, Richard. Every Wednesday night, they have "boys' night out." They go to an elegant restaurant in the neighborhood. Richard is allowed to order anything on the menu, no holds barred. After a brief conversation about Richard's school day, Joel tells Richard in great detail about his own day at the office—clients that gave him a hard time, office jokes, money problems of the world. He imagines that this is of great interest to Richard. Richard tells me otherwise, that he just listens attentively to humor his father, but he's really rather bored. And he'd rather just go for a hamburger.

Moira and Joel both need help establishing clearer boundaries and a better balance between "baby and me" if their children are going to become authentic and autonomous young adults. The required psychological arithmetic used to be very clear. As the old song goes, "Just Molly and me, and baby makes three." But today's parents are confused whether baby makes three, or two in the case of single parents, or whether "baby is me." Although parents across generations have always experienced some merging between themselves and their babies, especially in the early months, we will see how parents today suffer from a surfeit of such merging. We flounder at demarcating boundaries between ourselves and our children *throughout* our child-rearing years, and are hard pressed to give a clear answer to the question, "Who am I doing this for, me or my child?"

THE BALANCE BETWEEN BABY AND ME

The field of psychology entered the second half of the twentieth century with a new focus on the development of the self in society. A group of psychoanalysts, psychologists, and child development experts have centered their investigations around the question, "How does a baby become a whole and separate human being?"

Clearly influenced by the world around them, all of these professionals were reflecting the increased social emphasis on the individual self as a separate unit and as the locus of salvation in the face of a society in which extended family and community were quickly disappearing. We find the ultimate metaphor of the modern "individualized being" in the gripping image of the fetus floating alone in space in the 1960s movie *2001*, a huge box office success.

D. W. Winnicott, the British psychoanalyst, referred to the phenomenon of selfhood as the development of individuality.[2] Margaret Mahler, an American researcher and practitioner, called it the separation–individuation process, with the final developmental achievement being a clearly defined and separate self.[3] Heinz Kohut developed a whole new school of American psychoanalysis, which he labeled "self psychology," in which he posited that the very thrust of life is to develop a sense of self.[4] More recently, Daniel Stern took Kohut's theory further and proposed a developmental schema in which life is organized around the establishment of four different domains of a self.[5]

But unlike the fantastic *2001* baby, the self does not develop in isolation, floating in space. We find out who we are through our connections with the people closest to us, starting with our parents. The task for parent and child involves a dialectical process: The child must become distinct from others in order to connect successfully to those others.

In addressing the first side of the dialectic—becoming separate—a new focus on personal boundaries sprang up in the second half of the twentieth century. Both the professionals and the lay public began speaking of the boundaries between self and other, between parent and child, between reality and fantasy. It became common parlance to tell someone close to you, "I need my own space." In the culture at large, there was a fear of having one's own personal self smothered or snuffed out by a violation of personal boundaries. People were growing edgy about where they stopped and another person started. It was not always so clear.

That edginess then brought people right back to the second side of the dialectic—making connections. By the late 1960s, the American divorce rate began to skyrocket and the Peter Pan generation was looking skeptically at the potential entrapments of any kind of relationship commitment. But, over time, they discovered that the alternative is loneliness. If you're always running away from relationships and making sure that no one encroaches on your personal space, you begin to miss personal connections and can come to feel isolated and empty. Not feeling connected has made people as anxious as losing one's selfhood has.

So by the 1990s, we find the adults of childbearing age faced with a perpetual tension between establishing meaningful relationships on one side and protecting one's own individuality on the other. It is the struggle that the psychoanalyst Jessica Benjamin refers to in her book *The Bonds of Love* as the tension between assertion and recognition—a developmental dialectic, she argues, that we universally face. We want our self to be recognized and to recognize other selves, but not at the expense of effacing our own unique individuality for the sake of acceptance.[6] The present generation of parents, rumored to "want it all," is really a generation having a very difficult time negotiating this dialectic between separateness and connection, between assertion and recognition, between our own needs and others'. This tension extends to our relationships with our children.

MIRROR IMAGES

Most parents today are not consciously aware that they are struggling with tensions between their own needs and their child's when a baby arrives on the scene. Like generations before them, they speak in blissful terms of the uncomplicated feelings of baby love. A new mother reports: "Your complete mandate in the world is to hold this soft, cuddly, sweet little baby, and it feels so good, the way she fits against your body when you're nursing her. You get the feeling of a union you long for your whole life. You can let your boundaries down with a baby."[7] An obvious expression of mother bliss, it is also focused on her self and the things the baby can do for her. The baby is assigned special powers in this reflection not about baby but about self: "The baby transforms everything, every kind of mundane experience, into something magic." We see the overvaluation of the baby that Freud alludes to, but rather than pumping up the attributes of the baby, the mother is more intent on glorifying the magical experience that it provides for herself.

D. W. Winnicott wrote extensively about the parenting that would provide for the child the opportunity to grow into a healthy and whole individual with a firm sense of his or her own uniqueness. For that to occur, the parent, early in the child's life, has to be able to serve as a "mirror" to the small baby. When the baby looks up into the parent's face, the baby, still only weakly formed, is actually searching for a reflection of itself, through the parent's gaze, expression, and communicated focus on baby and all that baby is. The parent is to "mirror" back what that parent sees in the baby, imitating the baby's coo, smiling back when baby smiles, and so forth. Through that process, the baby begins to develop a consolidated sense of who she or he is, and is allowed, in Winnicott's terms, to "go on being," that is, to naturally unfold with her or his own unique qualities of self. As the child grows and matures and develops a better sense of where he or she ends and others start, the child will no longer be so reliant on the parent as a mirror, but will turn more to the parent as a distinct other with his or her own selfhood.

When one-year-old Jasmine wakes from her nap, Tony, her father, waits for her to begin humming her little tune to herself, and then hums it back to her. It is a simple tune, sung in E minor. If she wakes up fussy, he is sure to switch his tactic and instead rock her gently, murmuring, "Jasmine's having a hard time waking up today." Occasionally, when he's in a rush or just feels harried, he doesn't wait for her signals and just swoops her up and changes her diaper, so they can get on with their day. But he doesn't feel good about himself when that happens, and Jasmine doesn't much like it herself. Those times are few and far between, however, as Tony is committed to making his time with Jasmine as uncontaminated as possible by his own hassles and stresses.

As Jasmine grows older, Tony is not so keenly attuned to tracing her every move through a responsive gesture. But he never loses the ability to mirror Jasmine when he intuits that it is important for Jasmine to assert her own little self and feel recognized by him. When she tells him at age four that she wants to be both an astronaut and president when she grows up, he doesn't tell her that's an awful lot for one girl to be. Nor does he applaud and charge in with a great celebration of her grandiose fantasies. Instead, he sits by her bed and listens attentively while she tells him her dreams, reflecting back to her Jasmine's own excitement through his accepting look and by his encouragement to tell him her story. Tony's actions over time are exemplary of good mirroring.

If a parent, however, is unable to serve as a mirror, as Tony did, but instead imposes all of his or her own needs, feelings, and preoccupations, problems will ensue. Instead of looking up at the mother's or father's face and seeing a reflection of self, the baby will look up and find nothing but the other person. Counting on the parents' mirroring for help in finding out just who he or she is, the baby will be chagrined to discover only an imprint of the other person. This leaves the young baby to feel that his or her own self does not really exist; only the other person's is real. In order to survive psychically during a time when the baby is totally dependent on the caretaking adults, the baby is left with no choice but to accommodate to the parent's moods and needs, denied the opportunity to freely experience its own. Ultimately, the child will then develop falsely, always putting up a good front but never feeling safe to be a genuine and authentic person with feelings coming from within rather than being totally reactive to pressures from without.[8]

We see this alarmingly in our clinical work with young babies and their depressed parents. Over time we watch an infant's smiles and coos transform to a sedated, lackluster state of ennui as the infant looks up at the mother's or father's face and finds blankness instead of responsiveness, distraction instead of attentiveness, sadness instead of a joyful response to baby's smiles or coos. There isn't a parent in the world who doesn't on occasion look down on their young baby in such a fashion. But when it becomes a regular pattern, we watch babies not even old enough to talk distorting their own sense of being to adjust to the distorted mirror placed in front of them by their parents' inability to shake themselves from their own depressed state.

I do not want to give the impression that this is a problem confined to depressed parents. Letty was ecstatic when her first child came along. Herself an energetic and dynamic woman, she was accustomed to meeting the world with enthusiasm and optimism. As is so often the case, her new little boy, Drew, was of a very different temperament—low-keyed, somewhat slow to warm up. Every time Drew awoke from his nap she would dash in, pick him up, chortle to him, and jostle him on her knee. Often Letty would spontaneously run up and tickle Drew's belly or play three little piggies with his toes when he was lying laconically in his play pen. Already, by age one, Drew was "tuning out" to ward off the intrusions.

At age four, he told his mommy he wanted to be a nurse when he grew up. "Why would you want to be a nurse when you could be a wonderful doctor?" she replied, hoping to steer him toward more gender-appropriate choices, broaden his horizons, and bolster his self-esteem. Never did he get a chance to tell his own story about the wonderful things nurses did in the story his teacher just read, things that he, too, would like to do when he grew up. Regrettably, Letty was engaged in "not good enough" mirroring.

The "mirroring" concept is another way of expressing that being a good enough parent requires seeing your children as separate people and not putting yourself before them or imposing on them what you want them to be. To be a good mirror requires a careful and graceful balancing act between self and other: to bring all of your being to the experience, but only as focused on the child. I believe mirroring is a particular aspect of parenting mothers and fathers struggle with today. The new mother above who speaks of baby love gazes at her child and is filled with feelings about herself rather than her child. This does not bode well and may certainly be prime cause for a crack in the parenting mirror. The potential outcome is a reversal in which the child now becomes a mirror for the parent. Rather than giving the child back a reflection of the child's self, the parent anxiously seeks to find him- or herself through the child. If we are a generation that is floundering to figure out just who is our center, self or baby, it makes sense that we would be vulnerable to such reversals.

We are not the first generation to struggle with this. An experience from my own high school years remains indelibly etched in my memory. I was involved in a theater production. One of my dance partners, quite an accomplished performer, was herself the daughter of an ex-professional dancer. Her mother came to every one of our rehearsals. Finally, during a dress rehearsal, directly following her daughter's performance, my friend's mother lost all composure and ran down the auditorium aisle gleefully shouting, "She's just like me, she's just like me." We all stood gawking, amazed not that a mother would feel this, for I am sure many do, but that she would so openly express it. It was a jarring experience for me—the naked exposure of a mother's uncontained overinvolvement in her daughter and the unabashed wish for a clone. More disturbing was the outcome—my friend went on to have a "nervous breakdown" in her college years.

Michael, an eleven-year-old son of a divorced couple, returns a book of short stories that his father bought him because, while out with his mother, he found another one that was more complete and exactly what he was looking for. Michael tells his mother he is worried that his father will be angry with him for returning the book. His mother reassures him that, although his father sometimes does explode, he won't be angry at all this time, he might even get a kick out of it, because it will reflect that Michael is just like his father, who has an obsession about books. Michael is dubious, and with substantial trepidation he makes the phone call to his father to tell him he returned the book and to explain why. He comes back from the phone call beaming. Just as his mother predicted, his father was just fine about it, exclaiming, "Oh, good, you're an obsessive just like me." For Michael, there was short-term relief. But in the long run, Michael's own authenticity may be jeopardized as he learns that the way to win his father's favor, rather than his wrath, is to be a mirror for Dad.

In these two parenting stories, a generation apart, we find reverse mirroring, based on the parent's belief that the child reflects back a spitting image of who the parent already believes him- or herself to be, in the case of the book-obsession father, or to have once been, in the case of the ex-dancer mother. In Michael's story, his father's exuberance in finding a son who is just a chip off the old block is not a rare phenomenon but an all-too-common portrayal of parenting today.

Such mirroring reversals have become so commonplace as to be etched in no one's memory but simply absorbed as an expectable part of parent–child relations. They are no longer something to be gawked at, as I did with my friend's mother. In the mid-1990s, we read a by-line for a *Parenting* magazine column, "A father searches for himself in his newborn's face."[9] A contemporary mother describes her relationship with her young daughter with unabashed pride: "Allison may not give me the respect I gave my mother, but I never aspired to be like my parents. And already Allison wants to be an environmentalist *just like me*" (italics mine).[10] "Just like me" substitutes for "Look into my eyes and find *yourself* reflected."

But this is not the sole type of breakdown in appropriate parental mirroring that plagues mothers and fathers today. Mirroring problems also surface when parents project onto their children not who they actually are but all that they would like to be, if given a second chance. In 1993, Lucinda Franks published a provocative cover piece in *The New York Times Magazine* as she depicted "Little Big People," the "miniature adult" side of the kinderdult phenomenon. In describing the motivation of parents to create a generation of children sophisticated, entitled, and sometimes just a little too big for their britches, Franks explains that we, the generation of parents who came of age in the Vietnam War years, wanted to undo our own parents' foibles and "create the children we always yearned to be."[11]

If we stop to think about it, it is a tremendous burden to become for someone else everything that person had wished to be or wished to have had. As a child, I longed to have music lessons. I begged my parents, but they said "No," because I was already studying dance. As is the whim of many children, I promised myself that when I grew up I would never do that to *my* children. I grew up. I had children. I made sure they had the music lessons I had always wanted. The problem was that they hated music lessons; it was never *their* desire.

It is always easy to be a Monday morning quarterback, but if I could do it over again I would have made myself take a good, hard look at my motivation and behavior in foisting music lessons on my children. With the insight I now have about the dangers in the reversals in mirroring, I might have recognized that I was so caught up in correcting the disappointments of my own childhood that I failed to see my son and daughter as the individuals they were. Instead, I projected my needs as their desire. This is clearly one of those incidents in which I believe that bringing my deeper motives to the light of day would have been enough to check my tendency to intrude upon rather than facilitate my children's growth, at least in the area of music appreciation. If I could have curbed myself, they might even have *chosen* to take music lessons, at a time when the fancy hit *them*, not me.

It is not unfamiliar to hear adults complain that as children they always had to live for their father, or for their mother, and they were never free to follow their own star. We begin to wonder how commanding today's little "majesty, the baby" really is. We see a whole generation of children who are potential recipients of distorted mirroring. They may have parents who want their child not to reflect back an *accurate* image of him- or herself, but a *corrective* image of what the parents had wished for themselves. Either way, accurate or corrective, the mirroring reversal robs the child of a reflection of his or her own genuine self.

YOU ARE MY SUNSHINE, SOMETIMES

Along with reversals in mirroring, there is fluctuation in the meaning of a child in parents' lives. A colleague relates to me the story of a fifty-two-year-old mother who videotapes most of her five-year-old adopted daughter's waking moments. Stored in her computer are extensive files on her child's comings and goings, ups and downs. We could say, in accordance with the authors of *The Too Precious Child*, that this mother is indeed creating a precious person, one who is "too important, too special, too much the center of parental attention."[12] But then we find that this same mother has been away from her child for three weeks, and it may be several weeks more, to spend time with her own mother in another state. The daughter, when asked by my colleague to state three wishes, had only one: "to see my Mommy, I miss her." This mom needs help seeing the contradictions and wild swings in her behaviors and attitude toward her daughter: too central, not central enough. Home more, but glorifying less would be a far better middle ground.

The reality is that the situation of the overvalued child today has an underside. Children are videotaped, but then left for several weeks at a time. Fathers forget about them or desert them after a divorce. The overvalued child is also the overridden child. This is an important piece of the kinderdult phenomenon. Parents vacillate between the child as cherub and the child as miniature adult. They run back and forth between attending to their own needs and those of their child's. As they swing on this pendulum, the meaning of the child to them fluctuates in turn—first the child is everything, then the child appears to be overlooked. This is a big problem for both parents and children today.

In economic terms, children have become a liability, rather than an asset. They no longer contribute to the family income, as they did in the nineteenth century. They are no longer relied on to take care of their parents in their old age. They cost parents a great deal of money; it costs an estimated 171,000 to 265,000 dollars to raise one child in the United States.[13] The government offers minimal to no support in that process, in contrast to other advanced industrial countries. A century ago, couples had large families to provide more hands that could pitch in. Today, most parents are hesitant to have any more than two children because, in addition to the lack of time, they cannot financially afford a third or more.[14]

No longer an economic boon to the family, we need to assert children's worth in other terms. If we accept for the moment a phylogenetically based desire among the human race for procreation and progeny, it makes psychological sense that we will be drawn to assign meaning and worth to that endeavor. And then in purely social terms, with the shift from the *inevitable* to the *chosen* child, the tremendous drain on financial resources must be balanced by some other good reason for making such a choice, particularly in a society that creates such a fetish of dollars and cents investments as a guide for living. The best reason—the human urge to procreate, carry on one's name or blood, and contribute to the next generation—does not suffice on its own.

In the immediate sense, we see the child's worth in the love, the pleasure, the close connection that he or she will provide us. But as a long-term investment, there will be no financial returns. Instead, our payback will be a successful child who makes a name for him- or herself in the world and reflects back on the mother and father a measure of their own social and psychic worth.

But how does that translate into a child becoming a perpetual home video star but sadly missing her mommy in her long absences? One author and mother depicts the first half of the phenomenon as follows: "Members of my generation . . . gave new definition to the cult of child worship. When I was pregnant, one friend teased me for turning my apartment upside down and buying a king-size bed (big enough for three): 'You'd think you were preparing for Caesar.' " This mother described hanging her four-year-old son's drawings all over the house, eliciting a response from her son, "Mom, you'd think our house was the Metropolitan Museum of Joshua!"[15] She knows that in her investment in her child she has made him the center of the universe. Sounds like the overvalued child.

But if this same mother is representative of the statistics regarding the drop in contact time with children in this country over the last twenty-five years, she most likely spends a lot less time with her little Caesar than her own parents spent with her as a child, up to a forty percent reduction. And she is probably having shorter vacations with her child and eating dinners with him less than her own parents did with her as a child. Not because she is off having a good time, but because both she and her husband have paid jobs that keep them away from their home and their family. She may be off working to cover that six-digit figure that goes into raising a middle-class child today. This mother, like so many of her peers, may have made a conscious choice to have her child, but now ruefully finds that there's little time in which to raise him. In this respect, the child loses his or her centrality. Then the parent tries to make up for it by swinging back to the child as deity. And Joshua and *his* peers may have a high price to pay, with a total confusion between being the star billing at the Metropolitan Museum and a child with nobody home.

The child is center stage; the child is on the periphery. A mother reports that she has approximately ten thousand photographs of her four-year-old: "If anybody wants to know what's happening with my child, there is probably a picture that captures it." Like the mother with the video camera and voluminous computer print-outs, such obsessive focus on the child is definitely unnatural and unhealthy. But then we discover that it is not the mother, but the baby-sitters, who have shot all the film, at the mother's request. It is the way this working mother compensates for not having enough time with her child.[16] If she has been forced to miss her child's first steps, at least she can have them captured on film. Her child is very precious to her, but is too often known only through the lens of a camera.

The child is the parent's sunshine, the child is hardly more than a shadow. It is a lethal combination. Parents believe their child should be precious, but they experience limited access to the precious child they have chosen to have. Perhaps the child grows even more precious the more infrequent the actual contact becomes. Anna Quindlen, a columnist for *The New York Times,* poignantly articulates the tensions parents feel:

> Since I've made a decision to be away from my children for a considerable portion of most days, I've got to make my peace with a couple of plain realities. One is that I'm going to miss some good stuff. There will be lots of fun had, questions asked, significant moments passed when I'm not there. . . . I suppose I feel sometimes that I've substituted trying too hard for not trying hard enough and frankly, from a child's perspective, I'm not sure which is worse.[17]

They are both bad, whether the parent *chooses* to be away from the children or *must* be gone to earn a living. Why does this happen—trying too hard, not trying hard enough? If her children didn't mean so much to her, she wouldn't try so hard to make up for her absences by feverishly creating so many precious moments in her presence. It wouldn't matter. But if the children were really so important to her, would she or could she have found some way to be around her children more? This is a real problem of parenthood today: What is the meaning of my child to me? Who really is my sunshine? Myself or my child?

FOR BABY OR FOR ME?

A father whizzes by with his baby girl, sweat running down his cheeks, red faced and out of breath. Is there an emergency? Quite the contrary. He is out for a jog with his little one, who is safely strapped in her jogging stroller, a large, three-wheeled vehicle designed for baby to sit in as Mom or Dad runs behind. Why not kill two birds with one stone— expose baby to fresh air and the outdoors, and get a little exercise for oneself in the midst of a work-packed, no-time-for-leisure daily life? The experience may be great for Dad, or for Mom if she happens to be the aerobic stroller pusher for the day. Yet I wonder what it means for baby—seeing the world fly by at record speed during a time of life about which we fantasize so nostalgically as a lost era of timeless exploration and slow, pressureless pursuits.

Babies, like royalty, were meant to have a leisurely pace. Transport in expensive jogging strollers hardly provides that. Instead, we have babies on the run. Yet such strollers sell like hotcakes to loving, caring parents because they meet the needs of harried mothers and fathers with limited time for child rearing and with knowledge that the more they exercise, the longer they will live. How many parents have actually stopped to contemplate what the experience might be for their child?

At the same time, thousands of new mothers and fathers across the country are "sneaking" their babies into bed with them at night, probably some of the same parents who race their babies in jogging strollers by day. With the exception of La Leche League, the professional advice in this country is consistent: Keep the children in their own beds, from birth to maturity. In the words of our American child-rearing guru, Benjamin Spock, "I think that whenever a child crawls into the parents' bed, she (or he) should be taken back promptly to her own—just as often as she does it."[18]

• • •

Traditional societies see this as barbaric, pushing a young infant or child far beyond its developmental capacities and forcing a premature independence that can only be toxic.[19] So do many modern parents, despite what their pediatricians or child-rearing manuals advise them. Here is one instance where they do not heed the "wisdom" of the experts. Instead, they choose to sacrifice the marriage bed for the family mattress.

Such sacrifice may well serve to avoid sexual intimacy. In a culture where sexual desire appears to take a nose dive after the birth of a child, a child in the middle is certainly a better excuse than "Not tonight, dear, I have a headache." Taking a child to bed may also be a function of expediency, to avoid having to get out of bed at night to tend to baby. Already exhausted by a harried schedule of balancing work and family demands, parents collapse into bed each night depleted. To drag oneself repeatedly from bed to minister to the needs of a child in the next room when one quick tuck in the little space between Mom and Dad can buy minutes of sleep may certainly lure overworked parents toward the latter solution. Taking baby to bed may also reflect parents' desire to be the best parents they can be—parents taking baby to bed may genuinely think this is best for baby and prevents early trauma.

We can now see how we vacillate tremendously between seeing our baby as royalty to be catered to, as when we take our young charges to bed to prevent trauma, and seeing our baby only through the lens of our own needs, as when we race them through life in jogging strollers. Sometimes, even within a single act of ministering to our child, we are vacillating between child as center of the universe, child as a reflection of our own needs. Bringing baby to bed is actually a perfect example. A couple may firmly believe that their baby will thrive better and feel safer if they rebelliously buck Dr. Spock's advice and bring baby to their bed. But at a deeper level, they may be as strongly motivated by their own desire for physical warmth and cuddling. A couple may have consciously decided to grant the child's dependency needs rather than enforce premature independence, but the unconscious reason for bringing baby to bed is to assuage their own guilt that ensues when they deny their child *anything*. They may tell themselves or their pediatrician that they bring their child to their bed because they have put their child's best interest first, but if truth be told, it is because they are simply too exhausted to do anything else.

What we have here is a conflict between conscious thought, which speaks to our child's best interest, and unconscious motivation, which speaks more to our own needs. Almost any social interaction involves simultaneously doing something for both oneself and for the other person. We sit next to our child's sick bed for hours at a time because we love our child and know that our child is vulnerable and needs more of us when taken ill. At the same time, we do it because it makes us feel good as parents. There is no contradiction between the two motives; they complement each other nicely. The quandary for parents today is that more and more of their parenting experiences do not blend together so nicely. They so much want to be good parents, but the motives for self and for other may be in conflict. This creates great anxiety for parents, in which their unconscious and conscious selves work at odds with each other.

Let us continue with the example of parents taking their children to bed. Judy is one of those parents. Her child, Cecilia, is now three and still spends most nights sleeping either at the end of Mommy and Daddy's bed or right between them. She often starts in her own bed, but nightmares wake her and so begin her nighttime travels to her parents' bedroom. Judy thinks this is just fine, if that's what her child needs, but Mark, her husband, does not. With their sexual intimacy diminished and their sleep repeatedly disrupted, he wants to come talk to a professional.

Judy and Mark assume they are just caught in a disagreement about child-rearing philosophy. But in the course of our consultations, I learn that Mark is more generally upset about the lack of boundaries between Judy and little Cecilia. He doesn't think Judy really believes it's better for Cecilia to sleep in their bed; he thinks she has her own need to be a mother who never rejects her child. Judy takes issue and snaps back at Mark for always putting his own needs first. She accuses him of rationalizing that sleeping in her own bed would be better for Cecilia's independence training when what he really wants is a night of uninterrupted sleep with the possibility of lovemaking. He should have known that they would have to give that up for a while when they had children.

Judy and Mark are each trying to dodge their own anxieties about balancing their own needs against Cecilia's by casting the blame on the other person. To get out of this morass, I first had to disentangle the parents from each other by directing them to stay inside their own fences and stop flinging mud at the other person. I asked each of them to concentrate on looking into themselves, free associating about all the ways they felt when Cecilia showed up in their bed. From there, I worked with each of them individually to differentiate as to when they were looking through the lens of their own needs and when they were focusing on Cecilia's experience and Cecilia's developmental needs. In some ways this task of differentiation is as difficult as separating the blue from the yellow in green paint—the paints seem to meld into a new, inseparable color. We could think of my role as the color separator.

Indeed, Judy and Mark did have somewhat different philosophies of child rearing, coming from their different cultural backgrounds, but more central to their conflicts were their own internal anxieties about trying both to balance and to separate their child's needs and their own. Once they could stop faulting the other person and reclaim their own anxieties, it was uncovered that Mark was right. Judy had a need to never say no to her child, lest Cecilia reject her. This need interfered with her ability to send her child back to her own bed, even when deep in her heart she really wanted a night's uninterrupted sleep. And Judy was also right, Mark sometimes grew impatient with Cecilia and demanded that she "go with the program" and fit into her parents' adult lives, a demand that stretched Cecilia beyond her developmental capabilities.

One thing Judy and Mark did agree on was the desire to do what was best for their child. Having applied the "color separation" technique—which gave both Judy and Mark insight into the question "Who am I doing this for, me or the baby?"—they were ready to take action. Together, we came up with nighttime techniques to soothe Cecilia when she awoke and to bring her back to her own bed. As Cecilia was a child who had had irregular and disrupted sleep since birth (a phenomenon that may well be constitutional rather than parent induced), Mark, in particular, would have to grow more accepting of Cecilia's developmental sleep irregularities. This might mean many more nights of interrupted sleep, but just not in *his* bed.

And Judy would have to work on her own need to be the perfect mother who never said no and focus instead on the goal of helping Cecilia experience the success of getting through a night's sleep safely in her own bed.

WHOSE BEST INTERESTS?

In the balancing acts between self and other, parents often catch themselves estimating not what is *best* for their child, but what their child will be able to *tolerate*. "Having a baby-sitter three nights a week when I go to my graduate classes after work won't be the *worst* thing for my child. She really likes the sitter."; "Staying home alone with the door locked from 3 to 6 P.M. won't be *so bad* for him. He knows how to use 911."

To soothe their anxiety about tolerable versus best, parents may give one explanation for their actions, yet be governed by quite another motive. A mother with three children interviewed by *The Wall Street Journal* justifies to her children the good effect of her and her husband's active careers on the children's lives: "I think kids need some distance from their parents to grow. It's really important for kids to make mistakes, accept their mistakes and learn from them. I think a real plus of my working is that you children are learning to be self-sufficient and feel good about the decisions you make." But the children have another story to tell: "Sometimes we want to talk to her when we come home from school and we get kind of annoyed that she's on the phone. Also, even though she works pretty close, it's kind of hard for her to come home. If we were sick or something she could pick us up, but it would be hard." Her other daughter reports, "I remember when you came home for lunch with us, you'd be home for 10 minutes and then go back to work." This mother asserts that she and her husband "have made a big point of putting the kids first in terms of seeing that they're not being sacrificed because of our careers." Yet the children expose their feelings of deprivation. She reveals the powers of rationalization as she sees only that her career is good for her children, believing that she has, in fact, put her children first. It is hard for her to admit that she has also put *herself* first. The reality is that she has very much wanted a career, which is both admirable and justifiable, and that her children have both benefited *and* suffered from having two parents who are actively involved in their work but are not around very much.[20]

Other parents are well aware that in certain respects they are not putting their children first, but they feel they have no choice. They work long or off-hours not because it is their career decision but because it is a financial necessity. They are often forced to put their children in less than ideal child care situations. The attitude of their employers is not to put the best interests of workers' children first, but to get the most from their employees.

Several large corporations have established company-based child care for parents on the night shift. Children are brought to the center at the beginning of their parents' shift. In such arrangements, pre-school-age children are kept up until late hours of the night so that they will sleep the next morning and allow their parents the opportunity to sleep after their night's work. A journalist explains, "As businesses that operate late hours or around the clock begin to address employees' child-care needs to guarantee a stable work force, more and more such children are enduring disrupted sleep in institutional settings so that parents can hold on to their jobs."

The parents interviewed were not happy that their children were put to sleep every night by child care workers rather than themselves, but they have no choice. The older children complained of the fatigue and overstimulation of being exposed twenty-four hours a day to other youngsters when forced to combine a school day with a night child care schedule. As one mother of a four-year-old put it, "We have no life. There is something about giving your child a bath and reading stories and putting him to bed. It is so special. I miss the mama stuff."[21]

These parents are perhaps better off than the career parents who speak only of the benefits to their children of their work and child care arrangements. They know that the child care arrangements take a toll on their children, but the night center is a must if they want to keep their job. There is no self-deception. But at the same time, they, too, like the mother reported in *The Wall Street Journal*, will have to grapple with the guilt or anxiety of putting themselves before their child, a conflict that is especially poignant for mothers (vs. fathers), whose ascribed role is *always* to put the children first. Over time, they, too, may feel pulled to construct a belief in the virtues of this arrangement to assuage their parental angst in the impossible balancing act between baby and me.

At a conscious level we know that our role as parents is to try to put our children's needs before our own. We should have thoughtful regard for our children's ideas and feelings. We must recognize that a child is not an independent adult and is therefore in need of our ministrations and attention, even when we must sacrifice satisfying our own competing needs to do so.

The deeply internalized dictum of our generation, "If it feels good, do it," amidst a larger culture that does not laud self-sacrifice, presents us with a parenting dilemma. If it feels good, and we do it, it may be at the expense of our child's well-being. Sylvia Hewlett, the author of *When the Bough Breaks: The Cost of Neglecting our Children,* has a nice way of putting it—our children suffer from our tilting toward the self.[22] We are so absorbed with our own inner worlds and ambition that we generate an unhealthy trade-off between personal fulfillment and family well-being. The children pay by getting shortchanged on the intensive time required to create a home and raise children optimally.

The capacity to remain focused on the child's best interests is further impaired by the blurring of the boundaries that historically separated childhood from adulthood. Our generation entered adulthood in the age of Aquarius, with the dictum that no one should have to take on the responsibilities of adult society if they did not feel so inclined, whether they were eight, fifteen, or forty. I was reminded of the power of this "youth mentality" at dinner with an old friend. Seriously involved with a woman in her thirties, this forty-two-year-old man, a highly successful attorney, told us he did not know if he was ready yet to have a child. If not by forty-two, when?

We have emerged into adulthood during a period of history in which the children's garden has been replaced by the fountain of youth—"I can live forever as a young and vital person." Children are allowed to act older than their years, adults are allowed to act younger. Sometimes it is hard to tell the children from their parents. Melanie, age forty-one, comes to her parenting session in sweatshirt, jeans, and a baseball cap. Waiting for her appointment, she opts to plop herself on the hallway floor rather than choose a seat in the waiting room. She runs her own business with several employees. Her son, Calvin, is dressed in almost identical clothes. He, too, thinks he runs his own business—at age seven he thinks it should be his choice to participate in classroom activities or not; nobody should be the boss of him. He uses very large words and sophisticated language.

Because of the boundary diffusion between adulthood and childhood, we parents often find ourselves overly merged with our children's experience as we gleefully move back into the pastures of early life that we only reluctantly left in our passage to adulthood. Either we join with their cherubic experience or we elevate them to adult-like status. Either way, we experience them as being just like us.

The media has been quick both to reinforce and to exploit the Peter Pan sentiment among today's parents. In 1993, Volvo came out with this ad for their cars: "For all those who have a family but aren't ready to settle down." The text continues: "For all those who continue to be a kid, even when they have one. For all those who have their feet on the ground, but find a lot of neat things to do there. For all those for whom childbirth is the continuation of adventure, not the end. For all those whose kids tell them to turn down the radio. We present an automobile . . . for all the children who will be born this year. And all the children at heart they will be born to." Those of us from the professional middle class all thought we bought Volvos because they were safe cars that would protect our children from harm. None of that is mentioned in this ad. The appeal is to our own narcissistic pleasure. Ads are designed to sell by appealing to the psyche of their potential buyers. Volvo's advertisement is only telling us what we must now face: We are always in turmoil as to whether we are doing for our children or for our young-at-heart selves.

Bruno Bettelheim, shortly before his death, chastised American parents for creating this turmoil. In reference to mothers and fathers today told an interviewer, "All they want is little adults. That's why we have so many childish adults who only want to play."[23] In other words, parents want their children to be able to go off on their own so the self-centered parents can continue to frolic about, unhindered by the presence of a needy dependent in their lives. His admonishment to parents seems overly harsh, but Bettelheim accurately underscored not parents' culpability but their confusion: Are parents adults or children? Are their offspring adults or children? What's the difference anyway?

We are pressured by the projections from our own childhood. We are influenced by the culture of self-gratification. We are confused by the permeable boundaries between adulthood and childhood that pertain today. We are frustrated by the external exigencies, such as unbending workplace demands, that make it impossible to be the good parents we would like to be. All of this subterranean activity leaves us groping for the internal markers that could guide us in a graceful interplay between ourselves and our babies.

A mother and father seek out a consultation because their six-year-old, Samantha, is not "making it" at school. She shows no motivation to learn, is timid around other children, and would prefer to stay home from school altogether. She also has minimal tolerance for any kind of frustration, reduced to a pool of tears if her jacket will not zip on the first try. We find out that every night she sleeps in her parents' bed and always has. (How intriguing that this issue of the family bed keeps popping up in modern parents who are having difficulty separating their own best interests from their child's.) Her parents defend this practice, staunchly taking an antiestablishment stand that attacks Western culture for being individualist, isolationist, and independence crazed. They patiently remind the consultant of the many cultures where children and parents as a matter of course share a common bed, to no ill effect. Further, they say, we are one of the only "deviant" societies worldwide that forces children to sleep in isolation.

The therapist wisely reminds the parents in turn that their child, unfortunately, is not a member of any of those other cultures. Instead, she must be helped to negotiate her own culture, one which expects a six-year-old to leave home, sometimes traveling long distances, to attend school for several hours a day. To accomplish this, she must develop certain capacities for independence, a process that appears to be impeded by her parents' coddling and lack of encouragement for "age-appropriate" functioning, culture bound though these standards may be.

The therapist gently probes further and discovers the real reason for the child's long-standing presence in the parents' bed. The mother

• • •

has had a chronic fear of sudden infant death syndrome and continues to feel that the only way to assure the child's survival is to sleep right next to her. Even though six-year-olds *never* suffer from crib deaths, she is not taking any chances. There is enough risk and danger in the world as it is.

Finally, through some work with the therapist, both the mother and father are able to see that their seemingly nurturant behavior fails to focus on what their child really needs or even wants. Unwittingly, Mom and Dad had failed to facilitate the autonomy that Samantha needs to make friends and feel confident in the classroom. For the first time, with the help of an understanding professional, they are able to see Samantha in her own right, as a six-year-old child separating from home to find her own way in the world of peers and school. Samantha is soon sleeping in her own bed, and overcomes her school phobia, and life for all seems happier at home.

Samantha's parents mean well. If they were not so dominated by their own needs and anxieties, perhaps Samantha's six-year-old crisis would never have come to pass. Samantha's parents would have been able to move on, satiated with the genuine feeling of being at one with their child and ready to meet the new challenges of their child as a growing and separate person. Instead, they had become arrested in that early stage of parenthood in which the child's and parents' needs are experienced as merged. Only when they could sort through, "Who am I doing this for, me or Samantha?", could they establish better boundaries between themselves and their daughter and give her what she needed for her forward development.

DO CLOTHES MAKE THE PARENT OR THE CHILD?

The confusion about baby or me and the mirroring reversals and distortions that transpire are elegantly exemplified in parents' sensibilities about children's wardrobes. Parents get a kick out of seeing their tiny children dressed in miniature copies of adult clothes. A mother· explains, "Adult clothes for children are so cute, it's a temptation you can't bypass. I can't wait until I have some friends over for dinner and have him come downstairs dressed in a little Guess outfit."[24] What makes this such an irresistible temptation for a parent? What is this parent imagining that her friends will think and feel as her young son appears in his fine apparel?

The child in this moment is presented as a miniature adult, but in essence the bedecked little one is really much more a baby doll than a little man or woman, expressing the parents' affluence, taste, and fantasies. Like an inanimate doll, the infant or toddler has no volition or desire in his or her wardrobe choices. Instead, the baby is a helpless recipient of the parents' whims. The "miniature adult" dressing of babies calls to mind the great thrill that little children get when they dress their pet dogs and cats in their own baby clothes. The child turns the pet into a person; the parent turns the infant into a miniature replica of self. This sets the stage for a denial of the child's own individuality and separate status. The blurring between baby and me in clothing does not bode well for the child's establishment of authenticity as he or she literally becomes the parent's mirror.

The irresistible temptation to indulge in such designer togs for tots is driven by multiple forces. Foremost is the parents' desire to look in the mirror of their child's face and see their own selves reflected. That is why the child must be dressed as a small adult and not as a baby doll. Yes, the expensive, adult-like clothing can also serve as a status symbol, announcing to the rest of the world the disposable income one has to spend on one's child. But so could a hand-crocheted, white lace baby gown with embroidered socks to match. The choice, instead, of miniature tuxedos, jogging suits, or Nike running shoes for children who can't even toddle signifies a parent looking for his or her own adult image in the presentation of the child.

The choice also reflects the blurred boundaries between adulthood and childhood in our culture today. Phillippe Aries reports that in earlier eras of history no clear demarcations occurred between adults' and children's clothing. In more recent history, beginning with the Renaissance, a separate status of childhood evolved and clear markers of transitions from early to late childhood and then to adulthood were reflected in clothing styles.[25] In the early twentieth century, young American boys, for example, wore knickers, and moved to long pants only as they reached adolescence. Starting in the second half of the twentieth century, the clothing styles differentiating childhood from adulthood have been challenged. Children are not only allowed or even encouraged to wear clothes that in the past would have been the sole domain of adults; adults now also indulge in clothes historically reserved for the younger set. So we have boundary breaking in both directions—children dressing like adults, adults dressing like children. Ten-year-old Lauren borrows Mom's lace camisole, Mom borrows Lauren's oversized Oakland A's sweatshirt. With no adult–child boundaries in place, the parent is free to dress the child any way he or she pleases.

Lastly, it is not only parents' search for themselves in the reflection of their children that drives parents to create miniature selves by dressing children in adult togs. It also reflects the problem of merging, in which baby does not make three but is definitely "me." The child, when experienced not just as a reflection but as an *extension* of self, will be a prime candidate for being presented as "just like me." So that when the mother waits with excited anticipation to have her bedecked son appear before what she imagines will be the admiring eyes of her assembled guests, she is likely fantasizing that her friends' "Oos" and "Ahs" will be as much for her as for her baby—"I am you and you are me." This strongly drives her intense investment in having baby dressed just so.

Both the culture's and the children's response to this phenomenon of dressing tiny tots like adults is telling. From 1989 to 1993, articles such as the following have appeared in the American press: "For School, Children Want Adult Styles"; "Power Duds for Children: School Kids Seek Identity in the Togs They Choose"; "Showing Too Much Too Soon: Whatever Happened to Jumpers and Overalls?"[26] Children as early as the preschool years are rebelling against their parents' clothing choices and taking firm stands about how they themselves want to dress, and how they want to dress is as little adults. If the latest rock star is wearing it, they want it, too. This may be a symptom of children out of control—too much in a hurry to grow up, so defiant that parent–child clothing battles are starting earlier than first teeth falling out, so precocious sexually that they are allowed to dress like sexpots by age seven.

The dress-a-baby-like-a-debutante phenomenon has had its repercussions and is emblematic of the difficulties of differentiating baby from me. For many reasons, children today demand autonomy and self-determination at a much earlier age than in previous generations.

This is certainly an effect of the miniature adult half of the kinderdult image of childhood. Interesting, however, that children should choose clothing as one of their chief battlefields. No doubt we live in a culture where clothing is a social statement, and we very much reflect who we are by how we dress. But perhaps the children, in precociously choosing clothing as a battleground, are also rebelling against the earlier mirror reversal phenomenon in which parents, in their own self-absorption, got great pleasure in dressing their infants and toddlers in their own image. The children no longer want to be their parents' mirror but a reflection of themselves. Yet simultaneously they are locked into accommodating to the reflection given back to them by their parents, a reflection that begins in their earliest months of life, as they are decked out in miniature replicas of designer clothes. Thus, they will continue to adopt adult-like clothing, just not their own parents' style.

Rheema was adored by her mother. As a small child, Rheema's mother bought Rheema a closetful of Laura Ashley dresses and beamed with pride when little Rheema would waltz down the stairs in one of the dresses she had purchased. Mom had adult versions of many of these same dresses and glowed when the two appeared in their dresses together. Rheema loved her mother very much and basked in the pleasure of these shared moments. But then Rheema reached adolescence and realized that her mother was always trying to find a reflection of herself as she gazed at her young and beautiful daughter. Rheema cast off her dresses and lace tights and chose a wardrobe consisting of torn jeans and faded T-shirts. Now, in her early twenties, her wardrobe remains unchanged. She vows never to be seen in a dress again.

I do not think this is Rheema's genuine desire. She is still being reactive to her mother's pressures, staunchly defending her right to choose for herself. She is so busy defending herself that she is never free to follow her own muse regarding both clothing and, more significantly, life-style. If I had been able to work with Rheema and her mother when Rheema was a child, perhaps I could have caught her mother's clothing predilections as symptomatic of a distortion in mirroring and tried to help the mother correct this so Rheema could be recognized as her own little person rather than a reflection or extension of her mother. And Rheema, rather than becoming a lost young adult, could have found herself.

• • •

MOTHERS VERSUS FATHERS

It probably did not escape the reader's eye that the clothing stories were all from or about mothers, not fathers. Indeed, fathers do not obsess in the same ways mothers do about the wardrobe of their children. A child's physical appearance is certainly often used as a measure of a person's merit as a parent. But nobody has ever hurled the insult, "Your *father* dresses you funny," while the corollary, "Your *mother* dresses you funny," is a well-known, age-old way to "cap" on another person. In other words, it is not just any parent's merit, but a mother's, that is under scrutiny.

But deeper, inner forces are equally as important as social pressures in creating a gender divide. Mothers, more than fathers, experience their children as an extension of themselves. Couple this with the fact that clothes in our culture mean more to women than to men, and we can understand how a mother seeing her child well dressed will thrill in her own sense of stylishness. It has no comparable charge for the father. In this case, clothes make the mother rather than the man.

The gender difference in parents' investment in their children's clothing tips us off to a more general distinction between mothers and fathers regarding difficulties in distinguishing between baby and me and balancing one's own needs with baby's. The work of Nancy Chodorow first alerted us to the phenomenon that men and women have different personality structures and relational abilities, based on their own experience of being primarily raised by a same-sex parent, in the case of females, or an opposite-sex parent, in the case of males. Men experience themselves as more autonomous and separate. Women experience themselves as more connected and related to others.[27] These differences are empirically evident in the way men and women parent. My own work with shared parenting couples revealed that women indeed found themselves generally more merged or connected with their children, while fathers were able to keep more of a distance, recognize the line where they stopped and their child started. On the other hand, men had a tendency to become more narcissistically involved in their parenting experience, focusing not so much on what they could do for their child but what their child could do for them.

· · ·

When a baby cries, a mother feels her own heart weeping. A father can more easily say, "Well, that's baby's problem, let's just try to fix it." But when a father realizes how special he is in his child's eyes, he becomes elated, even jubilant, in his experience of himself as a loved and admired person. A mother basks in the experience, but incorporates it as an expectable part of mothering. Both fathers and mothers struggle with mirroring reversals and balancing acts between baby and me in different ways: A father is more prone to put his own needs on an equal par or before baby's or to substitute his own face for baby's, whereas a mother struggles more than he to delineate the lines of where she stops and baby starts and to remain separate from baby.

In their own way, both mothers and fathers grapple with the dilemma, "Does baby make three or is baby me?" Mothers more often grapple with overconnection, and fathers with replacing their own image for baby's. But we are all caught in a perpetual balancing act of weighing our own needs against baby's and discovering either that they do not always mesh very well or that they remain excruciatingly blurred or entangled. To ensure that our children grow up to be authentic and differentiated human beings, we need to remedy our relationships with our children by finding a middle ground between having them be "too central" and "not central enough." Only then will baby make three.

CHAPTER FOUR

· · · · · ·

Parenting by Guilt

When will I get a chance to enjoy my daughter?
. . . When will I have time to do more than
discipline her? Because I work . . . I was cheating
Rachel out of a "normal life." . . .
    After that night, it became even more difficult for
me to leave Rachel with anyone for even a few
hours when I wasn't working. . . . There was no
way I could leave my daughter—we spent so little
time together already.
                                      —REGINA DICKERSON[1]

We parent like Tarzan on a rope, wildly swinging from never being there enough to being there far too much. It is time to find the key to the following riddle: How does this generation of parents simultaneously get construed as putting their own needs first and accused of being overly focused on their children? The answer to the riddle is one word—*guilt*.

Guilt has a very specific definition in psychological theory: an anguished state of mind arising out of an internal conflict. It is a state of mind in which we seek to make reparations, trying to fix what has gone wrong and make it up to anyone we have hurt. There could be no better descriptor for the predicament of this generation of professional, middle-class parents who have gone after what they have wanted—career, money, happiness—sometimes at the expense of their children's well-being and yet who also act as if the sky is the limit for their children. These parents indulge their sons and daughters and cater to their children's every whim. They do their children's homework with or for them, they let the children throw terrible epithets at them. Then they turn around and leave their children for long periods of time, too long, while they complete a work project or follow their own muse. And all the while they are in a stew, never feeling at peace with what they are doing, either for themselves or for their children.

Pulled in two directions, they run in both directions at once trying to fix the problem—too much for themselves, too much for the children. This is what I call parenting by guilt, the most pernicious peril of parenting, one that requires our immediate attention.

A PARENT'S LAMENT

Spring 1990. Oakland, California. Two sets of parents come to my consulting office on two consecutive days. The first set, Sarah and Dan, have designed a rigorous program of after-school activities and lessons for their nine-year-old daughter, Amanda, because they believe this will be beneficial to her. Amanda didn't choose this and she has no desire to participate, yet Sarah and Dan feel she "should." But that is not why they have come to see me. They are concerned about Amanda's belligerent behavior. An only child, and highly indulged by both parents, Amanda is always "mouthing off" at home. She tells them they're the stupidest people she's ever seen. She tells them, "No way, Jose, you can go f—— yourself before I'm doing this garbage homework." Sarah, an energetic woman in her late thirties, leans forward and blurts out with a combination of awe, dismay, and admiration, "We could *never* have talked to our parents that way! How does she get away with it?"

A day later, the second set, Michael and Cynthia, appear for their appointment. Both born in the aftermath of World War II, they are a warm and affectionate couple, strongly bonded to their son and daughter. Yet they each work long hours and employ a series of baby-sitters to cover their children's daily needs. Every night there is a battle with Robert, their ten-year-old son, over homework. Every morning there is a battle with him about almost anything. They look exhausted and shell-shocked. Cynthia reports a dream in which a tidal wave is raging toward their house, threatening to sweep her away. She knows the tidal wave is Robert. Michael, a mental health professional himself, has done his own miniresearch. He has asked every adult he has seen in the past week whether their own parents had ever been involved in their homework when they were growing up. His finding: not a one. He muses, "We are the first generation that is so damned involved in our kids' work. We're all so highly educated and we want the same thing for them. But it's crazy what we're doing."

"It's crazy what we are doing." This is the unifying lament that ties together the parents of our generation who came from the middle classes. It does not matter if our children are one, ten, or seventeen. We emerged from our youth with a vision. If we talked to our children, listened to our children, took them seriously, and had lives of our own that extended beyond the perimeters of parenthood, we would avoid the mistakes of our parents and have children who loved us, were close to us, and yet were independent, confident, and well prepared to face the challenges of living. We did not want to live *for* our children, but *with* them.

We meant well, yet our vision does not seem to be working. Rather than feeling that we have reached higher levels of consciousness and relationship with our children, we find ourselves in turmoil. Instead of having children who feel listened to, we have children who occasionally take liberties and verbally abuse us. The vision was well meaning, but full of contradictions. Children don't want to be lived with, they want to be cared for. Our way out of the morass is to let go of the fantasy of living *with* our children in favor of a more realistic notion of ministering *to* our children in ways appropriate to their ages and stages. But we also have to have the requisite time to do this.

Maria is the mother of an eight-year-old. She promised herself that she would never tell Anna to just stop whining, like her own mother used to. Instead, she would let Anna have her say, let her express herself, let her know that she had Maria's welcome ear. That was the least Maria could do after Anna's long day at child care while Maria was away at work. On the way home in the car one day, they got into a huge verbal struggle that ended in Maria screaming at Anna. Maria was devastated that this had happened, that she hadn't had the patience, the maturity, and the respect for Anna to hear her out.

But hear her out about what? On the way home, Maria reminded Anna that she had to finish her scouts project this weekend because out-of-town relatives were coming next week. Anna protested that Maria had promised her she could wait until the next weekend. Maria said she never promised that, and it would be impossible, because their guests would still be in town. Anna insisted, "You did, you did promise, Mommy." Maria explained calmly and with compassion that she was sorry for the misunderstanding, but that in any case, the project still had to be done this weekend because the family would be otherwise engaged for the rest of the week. Anna escalated, now in tears: "But Mommy, you promised, you promised." Maria repeated what she said before, stressing the misunderstanding but also the present reality. Anna went off in a tailspin, screaming, "*Mommy, you're not listening*!" And so it went, back and forth for the entire ride home until Maria exploded and Anna got scared.

Maria came to me feeling terrible about the irreparable harm she might have caused Anna in the explosion. I reassured her that the psychological bruises sounded only temporary and not of monumental consequence, but that I could understand how she would not want to repeat this kind of interchange. Working together, we discovered that if she had not been driven by her vision of the good parent who always listens to what her child says and always acknowledges her child's feelings, this drama could have been curtailed. Maria needed to listen instead to an eight-year-old's need to be contained and helped to accept that life doesn't always go her way, even when a misunderstanding his occurred. It also helped Maria to know that eight-year-olds are renowned for being oppositional as they try their new wings of independence and separateness from their parents. If Maria had had those tools in hand in her car ride with Anna, she would have been able to register Anna's complaint about the miscommunication, hold to her request of Anna, and then say, "End of conversation."

Additionally, if Maria had not been so consumed by guilt that Anna had not had enough of her during the day, she could have tolerated thwarting or frustrating her daughter momentarily in the service of helping her child (and herself) get out of a psychological tailspin. So it is not just our visionary parenting but also the pressures that push us toward work and ourselves and away from our children that need to be confronted if we are to move beyond "It's crazy what we are doing." It doesn't help to make desperate attempts to patch the holes in the safety net of the good life that was to be our children's birthright and protect them from falls—holes we believe we've contributed to because of our long work hours or lack of availability. It leaves us frantically scurrying to compensate or make up to our children for all that we cannot provide them. Parenting by guilt substitutes for visionary parenting, and creates the profile of a generation of simultaneously solipsistic and indulgent parents.

PARENTING BY GUILT IN ACTION

Grace, a spunky, intelligent mother in her early forties, is perched at the edge of her chair during a family therapy session. Doug, her seventeen-year-old son, highly distraught, is finally able to verbalize his inner turmoil. As Doug speaks, Grace silently mouths his words, as if they are her own, so overinvolved that she actually loses sight of the fact that they are not.

Doug, a first-born son and the apple of his mother's eye, was a model child in his early years. But upon entering adolescence, his world came crashing in around him, as happens to more than a few teenagers these days. His school grades dropped; he began experimenting with drugs; whole days would go by with Doug never getting out of bed. The more he floundered, the more Grace swooped in to pick up the pieces and try to fix him. The more Doug's heartache surfaced, the more she felt a knife turning in her own heart. Her career suffered; her health failed. The more she did for him, the more her guilt propelled her to do, because in her mind she clearly had not done enough.

Grace was faced with a major family crisis, but she is actually no different than many parents today in her intense, seemingly merged relationship with her child. More prevalent among mothers than among fathers, it was nonetheless one of the major findings of my shared parenting study that men and women who equally share the care of their children *both* have a propensity to be overinvolved with their children when they are with them.[2]

Taking to heart the new dictum of "quality time as an antidote to absence of time," parents try to make sure that every waking moment of the child's life in the parents' presence is filled with stimulation, fulfillment, and access to a parent's undivided attention. In shared parenting families, when both parents are home together, particularly at the end of a work day, rather than spell each other in their parenting responsibilities, they adopt an all-hands-on-deck approach to parenting. Four hands, rather than two, feed baby. Two players, rather than one, offer themselves as gamemates in a Candyland game. Mother and Father both listen to daughter's new piano piece, even if it means leaving the soup to boil over. I call this "wall-to-wall" parenting and believe it is one of the potential pitfalls of the shared parenting arrangement, exposing the child to a kind of emotional suffocation.

Wall-to-wall parenting is not unique to shared parenting families. Granted, there are still many absent fathers who partake little of family life or leave mothers totally responsible for the "second shift." But as I observe friends and family, take stock of my clinical practice, review other research findings, and follow the reports and portrayals of the family in the popular media, it is clear that parenting today among the American middle class includes an intense level of involvement in both the outer and inner lives of their children. *The Wall Street Journal* cites a survey finding by the Roper Organization that adults in the 1990s who have children seven to seventeen years old report doing far more things with them than parents in the mid-1970s said they did: "Simply put, parents today feel more strongly about being parents than was true over a decade ago."[3] This in spite of the fact that both mothers and fathers have less time in which to parent.

Parents sit every night with their children to do homework. They sign their children up for lesson after lesson and devote days of their own time interviewing prospective instructors to make sure they find the best for their child. If Sally has a fight with her friend Joanna, her parents do not stop at exploring with Sally what happened, helping her find a solution, and soothing her hurt feelings. They reach for the phone, dial Joanna's parents' number, and bring all four parents into Sally and Joanna's problems. Mothers may be doing this far more than fathers, but fathers are not exempt.

From a child's point of view, there is no breathing space to be alone, to negotiate one's own problems, to discover one's own solutions. Children can soon rely on parents to do everything for them and grow to expect that everyone will attend to them in the same focused way—teachers, child care providers, other relatives, and even friends. That is why some children of wall-to-wall parents have such a hard time in school, even with a small class of fifteen children—they expect immediate recognition and attention from the teacher, no matter how harried or busy that teacher may be. Why not, given that their parents seem equally harried at home, yet still don't miss a beat in catering to the children?

The solution seems obvious. Keep some of the hands off and give the children some breathing space. That is, however, easier said than done, for the guilt that drives such parenting behavior is so deeply rooted, so unconscious, and yet so active that we are often unable to get a grip on ourselves. I propose that if we can learn both to recognize and to manage our guilt, the more appropriate parental behaviors, including a more moderate dose of attention, will fall in place.

First, we need to know the guilt when we see it. It not only manifests itself in wall-to-wall parenting, it also shows up in this generation's incredible indulgence of our children, both psychological and material. Taken aback by the material indulgence of today's sons and daughters, a colleague tells me about her grown stepson and his daughter, Molly. Molly is one of those children with more toys than a toy store, and a separate bow, socks, and accessories to match each of her many dresses or play outfits. Like Maria with Anna, Molly's parents make every effort to listen to their six-year-old daughter, take her thoughts and feelings seriously, and treat her like a whole person in her own right. But somehow this well-meaning effort takes a wrong turn and translates into no responsibilities being demanded of Molly, whether it be to pick up her toys or help out on a family task. Yet almost every one of Molly's requests is met unconditionally. If Daddy is taking her to bed, but she prefers Mommy, she gets Mommy. If she wants to stop dinner to organize a group song, her wish is fulfilled, even if it means interrupting both dinner and an adult conversation.

Maureen, the mother of a nine-year-old, calls to tell me that she and her daughter are going to visit her ex-in-laws in Chicago. Her ex-mother-in-law has just called to say she would like to take them out to a nice dinner when they come, but only if Celine, the nine-year-old, will dress accordingly in a dress or upscale pants outfit. Maureen is in a stew, and very angry at her in-laws. She explains that she has a policy of letting Celine wear whatever she wants as long as it's clean, and that she hasn't placed dress demands on Celine for at least four years. No matter what quirky turn Celine's dress habits take, Maureen gratifies them. They usually take the form of undersized crop-tops, oversized T-shirts, and torn leggings. She imagines the grandmother's request will send Celine into a rage. Maureen is thinking of canceling the trip, one she herself had been looking forward to, because she feels her mother-in-law is being so unfair to Celine. She thinks better of it, but when the trip finally comes, Celine boycotts the dinner and demands the grandmother get her a baby-sitter rather than suffer the indignity of wearing clothes appropriate for the occasion.

Surely, these highly indulged children must come from a different set of parents than the ones who leave their older child with a key and a frozen dinner while they attend business dinners; bring their children to quiet supper clubs because that is where they, the parents, want to eat; or pressure their child to be perfect for *them*. No, quite the contrary. Molly is dragged to all her parents' dinner parties. Celine has had to accommodate to an ever-changing cast of men who have become her single mother's beau of the month.

Self-centeredness and an internalized belief that if it feels good, do it, can account for the self-indulgence. Pressures of work, career, and lack of time to get everything done can also dictate putting oneself before one's child. The swing toward overindulgence or overinvolvement then becomes a compensatory reaction. This is the essence of parenting by guilt. It plagues parents with a perpetual feeling of doing nothing good enough and creates the crazy picture of parents too focused on themselves and too focused on the children.

Work life is the key *external* factor in parenting by guilt. Trying to be a good enough parent in the context of present American job structures just isn't working. At the threshold of the last decade of the twentieth century, we began to see ripples of protest against workdays that leave children alone and parents away from their children for long hours. In 1991, Juliet Schor reported in *The*

Overworked American that, for the first time since such surveys had been conducted, a majority of Americans had been reporting that they were willing to relinquish even current income to gain more personal and family time.[4] In 1990, *The Wall Street Journal* printed an article titled, "Careers Start Giving in to Family Needs." Reporting that the "workaholic generation is working to put its family back on track," the authors explain that "the drive is especially evident for baby boomer women in their 30s and early 40s who've had fewer and later-born children, and now want to invest as much energy into their progeny as their deals."[5]

It is not only women, but men, too, who long for a better balance between career and family. A 1990 survey conducted by the *Los Angeles Times* indicated that forty percent of fathers and eighty percent of mothers reported they would quit their jobs if they could afford to raise their children at home.[6] Although this is still quite a large gender gap, it is notable that such a large percentage of male respondents would admit to even a *fantasy* of staying home to raise a child. A 1990 *Time/CNN* survey found that when asked about their lives and priorities, eighty-nine percent of the five hundred people polled said it was more important these days to spend time with their families.[7] When an investment superstar left his high-powered Wall Street position to spend more time with his seven-year-old daughter, he received more than a thousand letters from the general public expressing support for his move.[8]

In the meantime, however, the vast majority of parents do not have the luxury of quitting their jobs. Further, reported attitudes and actual behaviors are not always consistent. Parents report that they would like more time with the children. Yet if actually given the opportunity to cut back or quit their job, these parents might act otherwise. The need for security and the importance of work in their lives might well take over if faced with an actual choice. But they also know that the present arrangement is not a viable one for good family life, whether they act on that knowledge or not.

The swell of young people coming up right behind these parents speak even more loudly about the pull toward family over work. A woman who runs a job placement office in a local graduate business school is astounded by the change in feelings of the students in their late twenties, both men and women, who have come to her in recent years for advice and counseling. "Yuppiedom" is dead. Male and female students alike now face a dilemma. They spurn the fast track. They want to know how to pick a job that will allow them time to raise a family. The men accept that they will have working wives. They accept that they will be involved in child rearing. Students have stalwartly refused to sign up for interviews with some of the major megacorporation recruiters on the grounds that work conditions would be inhuman and grueling. They look at the work grind and lack of family time of men and women ten or twenty years older than themselves, and shout in loud protest, "Not for me."

Juliet Schor's findings corroborate this shift: "Both men and women, particularly younger ones, are adopting new expectations about family and career. They are overturning the assumption that men are responsible for breadwinning and women must take the second shift—trends that point in the direction of more balance between work and family."[9]

But the folks already caught in the parenting grind do not recognize that they too could have the choice of pronouncing, "Not for me." They are caught up in the current, which makes them feel that they *have* to make a certain amount of money if they are to feel comfortable and secure in themselves and give their children a good life, from now through their college years. As the dollar keeps dropping in value, the current only grows stronger.

I have two dear friends nearly buckling under the load of three children and two very time-consuming, demanding jobs. They are presently in debt, with house payments, school payments, and attempts to build college trust funds for the children. Their middle child is showing significant signs of stress, both at home and at school. Her teacher has called them in for a conference to express her concerns. Only the cries for help from this little girl have gotten my friends to stop and think that they may have to jump the fast track to heal their child's present suffering. Before that, they just felt that they had to keep going and going for everybody's ultimate happiness and well-being. The problem was that no one was happy and their well-being was questionable. Fortunately, they are both genuinely committed to the best interests of their children and they are both in professions where they can control their work hours and cut back, and that is what they intend to do, even if it means less disposable income for lessons, trips, and private schools.

Caught in such a current, what do most parents do? They don't always have the job flexibility or choices my friends do. Stop for a moment and reflect on your own feelings or imagine the feelings of any mother or father who has a full-time, demanding job and children, with little time to spend with them. Particularly if you are a woman, you will feel incredibly guilty that you are not fulfilling your parental responsibilities. Cultural norms may have made room for women in the workplace, but in no way has it substantially altered its ideology that every child needs the care and concern of a *mother* to grow up healthy. Given the recent emphasis on the comparable importance of fathers in their child's development, men are no longer exempt from this guilt, which used to be the sole terrain of women. Although they suffer from only a very mild case in contrast to the women, men, too, have begun to feel the pangs.

Take it a step further. Your child brings a note home from school saying her math performance is substandard. The note instructs you to please devote additional time helping her memorize her multiplication tables. It cites the average amount of time parents in the class have been working with their children on math. Implication: You have not done enough. You learn that you are at fault if your children are stressed because you are not providing a relaxed enough home life. You yourself have not relaxed in several weeks, what with work, parenting, and household responsibilities.

The family magazines and how-to-manuals reassure you that if the quantity of time you have with your children is not enough, you can make it up with "quality time." Time that you put aside just for your child. Typically, these scarce moments with Mom and Dad are filled with whirlwind activities designed to bring pleasure to the child. The other kind of time—filled with the everyday rhythms in which child and adult learn to share a space comfortably, some of it just quiet "nothing" time, some of it when a parent is preoccupied, and some when a child would be best left alone, is rare indeed.

Even when time is scarce, "nothing" time may sometimes be better than "whirlwind" time—more beneficial to the mental health of both parent and child. Amy and Fred come to my office to consult about their six-year-old son, Felix. Both of them work very long hours, leaving only a few squashed hours at the end of the day for the family to spend together. Amy is angry with Fred that on his time with Felix he just lets Felix go into his room and do whatever he wants. Mom feels Fred is being neglectful, and that as they have so little time with Felix, the least they can do is to fill it with fun activities and to *relate* to him. That's what she always does. Fred is irritated in return, protesting that Felix *likes* his time alone in his room more than anything. It takes some mediating skills on my part to calm the waters between Amy and Fred, get them to see each other's point of view, and then focus on what it is that Felix actually wants and needs, along with what they want for Felix. There is nothing wrong with the "nothing" time, Amy comes to see, but at the same time Fred acknowledges that in his "quality time" with his son, he might help Felix, who is quite a loner, by spending some time with him rather than allowing Felix to retreat into himself. Mom needed to provide more "nothing" time, Dad more "relating" time.

But even if we substitute or balance whirlwind time with nothing time, deep in their hearts parents know they are being sold a false bill of goods. As with any relationship between people who love each other, you have to take the time to make it happen. And parents do not have that time for their children. So they are forced to cram all their parenting into a thimbleful of available moments. Guilty that they have been away at work all day, they want both to assuage their guilt and to reassure themselves that their children are not angry at them when they come home. They worry that their children have suffered. And because they are part of a generation who does not believe that they or their children should ever have to suffer or that any good could ever come from suffering, their guilt escalates and they offer reparations. They want their child's acceptance, a signal that they have not done anything so terrible by having been away so much. They do this by creating a child's fairyland—no rules, no household demands, prince or princess for the evening.

"We ask so much of them already (by our absence), how can we possibly ask any more of them (in our presence)?" This is the guiding principle that informs mothers and fathers in their parenting by guilt.

It is in this fairyland that mothers and fathers will indulgently substitute *things* for time. It is Molly's room filled with wall-to-wall toys and floor-to-ceiling clothes. Certainly many a shopping spree is a form of conspicuous consumption so all can see how the parents are prospering. But when we see so many parents who are just scraping by who nonetheless make sure that their child has all the latest Nintendo games, because "that is the least I can do," we are also seeing parenting by guilt in action.

If guilt is an anguished state of mind arising out of internal conflict, the key *psychological* force that fuels this conflict for parents today is the golden rule with which we were brought up: the pursuit of happiness. Often, it is hard for us to shake the golden rule, even when we become mothers and fathers. We see it in the fathers who leave a fine job in one state to opt for a better one in another state, coming home only on weekends, because of their desire to better their career. We see it in the mothers who celebrate in the opportunity to go back to school and pursue a career on their own, often with little support from their husbands, but with the trade-off of putting their children in ten to twelve hours of child care a day. We see it in the fathers and mothers who leave a marriage that might have been salvaged in pursuit of greater happiness, despite the havoc the marital dissolution might wreak on their children. I am not talking about the parents who are terminally at war with each other, where a release from constant marital turmoil through divorce can well be an emotional boon to the children. I am speaking of couples with some general malaise or discontent that might be worked out if given a chance or even accepted as part of the reality of imperfect marital life. These are often the parents that end up in my own or someone else's consultation room, troubled by the stresses surfacing in their children.

"Finding oneself" or "pursuing one's dreams" can crash head on with nurturing a child. It does. And at a deep level we know it. In therapeutic work we differentiate between behavior that is "ego syntonic" and behavior that is "ego dystonic." Ego syntonic behavior causes us no internal conflict. It feels in harmony with the root of our being and our deepest desires and needs. That does not mean that it is healthy behavior, only that it causes us no pain. An example would be the divorced mother who looked at me blankly when I explained to her that her four-year-old son was deeply suffering from the lack of time he had with his mother. She responded, "What's the problem? Don't most working mothers work from seven in the morning to eight at night? Are you trying to guilt trip me?" Ego dystonic behavior is behavior we engage in but are troubled by, behavior that makes us feel that we don't like that part of ourselves or wish that we behaved differently. It is the mother who sits at work agonizing that her child is spending so many hours in child care, bothered that she may be being less than a good mother by having chosen an inflexible job with such long hours.

It is my assessment that most of us are suffering from ego dystonic parenting. We do not like ourselves for the way we parent. We are conflicted, not complacent, about the precarious balancing act between our needs and desires and our child's. The golden rule of the pursuit of happiness haunts rather than helps us.

To feel better about our parenting, and indeed, to parent better, we will need help managing our guilt and recognizing that it is not an all-or-none phenomenon—there is room for both ourselves and our child, even when there is precious little time in which to parent. But we will have to be willing to give something up and confront the limitations of our golden rule. We can't have it all, nor can our children. And life is not simply about happiness. It is happy, but it is also sad. It is fulfilling, as well as frustrating. It provides pleasure, but also metes out suffering.

Regretfully, my dear friends with three children may have to forestall reaching the pinnacles of their careers, but by pulling back on work they will have the payoff of an emotionally healthier daughter. Their daughter's distress signals will also afford them the opportunity to move beyond parenting by guilt. First they will be forced to feel the guilt acutely as they look at the crazy balancing act between doing too much and too little that is harming their child. Then they will engage in genuine repair, rather than some manic frenzy to fix their daughter's anxiety through wall-to-wall parenting or overindulgence. The reparation will involve providing their daughter (and their other children, too) a more laconic life with more time with their mom and dad. And if the psychological theory about guilt is correct, this true reparation will alleviate the guilt and move them beyond the underlying conflict that was causing it—I should have it all; my child should have it all.

PARENTING BY BEEPER

Parenting by guilt is actually a matter of time and place. When with the children, parents place the children at center stage. All eyes are on them. No wish is denied, no demands made. Parents give "too much." But that does not negate the other reality that parents are spending so much time away from the children in other pursuits. During those times, parenting falls into the category of "too little."

I have come across an intriguing attempt by well-meaning parents to try to correct the problem of not being *with* the children enough: *parenting by beeper*. Many working parents today carry electronic beepers so that their child can reach them during an emergency. This is a very practical solution for parents who are not always near a telephone and for children left alone after school for extended hours. But it also has a deeper meaning. If parents can't be there in person, at least they can be totally available by electronics.

Catherine is a professor at a local university. She carries her beeper so that her nine-year-old daughter, Barbara, can reach her, but has instructed Barbara to call only in a dire emergency. Otherwise, she should contact her grandfather, who is almost always readily available and willing to help. Catherine is in the middle of a lecture. Her beeper goes off. Catherine interrupts her lecture and dashes to a phone, heart pounding, terrified of a catastrophe. It's her daughter. Barbara's at school and she just doesn't feel well. Why didn't she call her grandfather like she's supposed to? Catherine chides. She just felt like talking to her mommy, Barbara retorts. Catherine is exasperated, her lecture interrupted, her space at work violated. Ironically, when she returns to class, her freshman students, having just left home themselves, applaud her willingness to carry a "mommy beeper" and have no complaints about her interrupting the lecture for her daughter's needs. Indeed, Catherine still keeps her beeper, and there will probably be a lot more calls like this one.

Melissa, just a year behind Catherine's students, is now a senior in high school. Her mother is a mental health professional. Melissa is furious at her mother for *not* wearing a beeper, even though her mother has an answering machine and checks her messages hourly. Melissa feels she can't talk to her mother whenever she wants. She should be able to—what if she needs permission to go off with a friend to San Francisco, or what if she had a particularly rotten day at school? Melissa plans to keep working on her mother until she agrees to get a beeper. That's the least she can do for her daughter if she's going to be away at work all day.

We see children expressing that they do not get enough of their parents, particularly their mothers. (It would be interesting to document how many beeper fathers there are compared to beeper mothers). At the same time, in Catherine's choice in wearing a beeper and Melissa's demand that her mother purchase one we see a collapsing of too little and too much parenting. Too little in that parents are not around very much with their children, too much in that there are no barriers between parent and child and children are given the license to demand their parents' attention *whenever.* I believe this is one of those frantic attempts at reparation for parents' guilt. It would be better substituted by a genuine increase in parents' physical availability and a healthy reduction in the amount of overindulgence we deliver to our children that leads them to expect "Mommy and Daddy on demand."

PARENTING BY GUILT AND THE KINDERDULT

Parenting by guilt is closely related to the modern child, the kinderdult. Specifically, parenting by guilt is responsible for shaping and reinforcing our new split image—half cherub, half miniature adult.

Even with beepers, when a parent is away at work or engaged in other pursuits, he or she will be comforted by the belief that children can make it on their own, without the ministrations, attention, or protection of the mother's or father's presence. To tolerate the guilt about being away from their children for so many hours a day, parents have to call forth some image of the child that will reinforce this belief in the child's independence and assuage the guilt. The miniature adult half of the kinderdult is the perfect image. It elevates the child to the status of someone who can handle waiting eagerly at the day care door at six o'clock in the evening, carrying a key and letting him- or herself in after school, or being a solo microwave chef three evenings a week. That miniature adult status can also delude parents into assuming that children, as miniature adults, will be partaking in the same pleasures as parents do when engaged in the pursuit of their own happiness. Child, like parent, will do fine with dinner parties, late-night hours, jam-packed schedules.

But holding on to an image of the child as a miniature adult is only a temporary fix, another frantic attempt at reparation. The guilt about not being there enough or providing enough eventually breaks through, and the parents open their eyes and see a child who is weak and helpless, in need of their care and attention, the cherub half of the kinderdult. Rather than the miniature adult who can handle whatever a mother or father can or whatever is necessary in the parents' absence, the parent now vacillates toward the tiny child in need of care and protection. Our guilt mingles with our perception of the cherub to construct the fairyland of the "second shift." If we can't shield them from the vagaries of the outside world in our absence, the least we can do is create a totally conflict-free sphere at home for our poor babies.

When Rebecca was one year old, her parents placed her in group day care five mornings a week while they worked on their PhD dissertations. Rebecca did not take easily to this arrangement. Every morning she clung to her parents when they dropped her off. All morning she whimpered periodically for her parents and refused to take off her little blue fuzzy jacket, regardless of the heat of the day. Often her parents would find her red-faced, sweating, and subdued when they came to pick her up. But they were inclined to think that this arrangement was good for Rebecca, that over time she would get used to it, and that it was beneficial for toddlers to be with their peers and develop relationships with other adults, rather than hanging around the house all day. They truly believed that her competence was steadily growing, even though the little blue jacket never left her shoulders. In the meantime, Rebecca's parents finished their dissertations.

Yet every night from ages one to six Rebecca protested if her parents left her sight for even a moment. She wanted not just one, but both parents there. She wanted her parents to entertain her, she wanted her parents to enjoy her entertaining them. She also woke them up several times a night, to comfort her and keep her company. They complied, for they believed that, by night, their daughter was sensitive, of a delicate temperament, and in need of extra ministrations. They saw no contradiction in their perceptions of Rebecca-by-day and Rebecca-by-night.

Many years later, with Rebecca now a grown young woman, her parents look back and wish they had done it differently. They recognize that her early child care program was too stimulating for her and that, given her temperament and emotional needs, she would have done far better with a single provider in her home. They wish that they had engaged her in more of the "nothing" time to which I referred earlier, helping her to find her own internal resources. They both agree that they were too lax on her nighttime wakings, and should have been firmer in communicating to her that nighttime was for sleeping and daytime was for working through problems. I can attest to how strongly Rebecca's parents feel this, because they happen to be myself and my husband. As working parents, we wish that we could have gotten a better grip on our guilt and not felt we could make everything up to our child by letting her be queen through the night. If we could have done that, it would have allowed us to put Rebecca in better focus. It is always so much easier to catch ourselves after than before a fall, but if we can offer such hindsight to others as foresight, it might help mothers and fathers think twice and check themselves on their tendencies to parent too much and too little while vacillating between perceiving their child as miniature adult and as cherub.

We pressure our children and feel neglectful and then coddle them to compensate. When pressuring, we see the miniature adult before us. When guilt-ridden, we see the tiny cherub. We ourselves are left reeling from the wild swings between our perception of the child as adult, the child as infant. And that is how we come to feel that "It is crazy what we are doing." It is not only crazy, but as with Rebecca's parents (myself and her father), it prevents us from hearing what our children are communicating to us and from tuning in realistically to our children's capabilities and needs and providing for them appropriately.

We do not feel guilty about our wild swings between parenting too much and parenting too little. It is just the opposite. Our guilt is what *causes* the swings. The swings are the symptom, the guilt the disease. That is why the ultimate solution is to attack the guilt—if we don't take care of the underlying disease, the symptoms will simply keep reappearing or will show up in new ways.

Whether we are away or at work or frantically trying to make the most of our limited hours with our children, we are always caught in the midst of the riddle—too much or too little parenting? There are two very specific arenas in which parenting by guilt is most poignantly experienced, both by parent and child. The first is the parents' thoughts, feelings, and actions about their children's achievements in life. The second is the parents' struggles to provide discipline and guidance to their children. In the next four chapters, we will address these two areas.

CHAPTER FIVE

· · · · · ·

My Toddler, the Doctor

We all tend to think our children are the most brilliant, most beautiful, most extraordinary on the planet. And we all worry that we may miss some facet of their specialness, that through oversight we may neglect to bring out the best in them.
—MICHAEL SCHWARTZMAN[1]

Mothers and fathers are now able to chart their child's development even before their child leaves the womb. The sonogram videotape has become a new source of home entertainment in households all across America. Mom- and Dad-to-be, relatives, and close family friends sit in front of the TV cooing over the movements, shape, and form of the unsuspecting little human being in the making. Already the fetus has moved beyond an abstract concept or hallucinatory vision to a viable and visible person. If prenatal testing identifying the sex of the baby has been performed, parents can even begin to formulate concrete gender expectations of their little man or little woman. And so the race begins.

Parents want a perfect child, and now they have to figure out what that is and how to get there. Before our children are born, we dream of their future successes. Then when they come, we feel compelled to shape them in that direction.

In my own childhood, the joking reference in Jewish culture was to "my son, the doctor." First-generation American Jews recognized that their sons' best chance for success and status in the United States involved sending their boys to medical school. A complementary message was sent to daughters: "Find yourself a nice doctor to marry." Times have changed since then. Impending reforms in

American health care suggest that medicine may not be the most lucrative or prestigious occupation for a young adult to pursue. Many other avenues of success have opened up to Jewish people. But the sensibility that I knew from my own background that children should be high achievers and reach for the top is not only entrenched, it has spread to every corner of American society. The only difference is that the age of achievement is set much earlier and the parental sensibility "My son, the _____" is now generously extended to daughters. And so we have, "My toddler, the doctor."

THE RAT RACE

A mother and father came to me for a consultation about their one-year-old. The presenting problem was the choice of a preschool for their infant two years hence. I found out this information on the phone, knew it to be a little unusual, but was intrigued to learn more about the real issues for this family. The mother entered the consultation room tense and drawn; the father seemed a bit perplexed. The mother explained: She was terribly concerned that she was not going about the search for a preschool program for her daughter in the right way and wanted some counsel. She had heard from others that one needed to begin the process well in advance, given the limited number of spaces for a swelling population of children. Breathlessly, she went on, "If Arielle doesn't get into the right preschool, she won't be in the right feeder for the good grade school, and then she'll be left with a permanent handicap when it comes to high school and college." Mother began to quietly sob, "I don't know what I'm doing. I've never been a parent before. And I hate all this pressure. And I think it's terrible, for me, for my child. But I can't escape it, because everyone else is doing it, too, and I don't want my child left out in the cold." Father remained silent, as men are often wont to do in such consultations, worried for his wife and confused about his own feelings on the matter.

In the immediate sense, this mother needed reassurance that everything she was doing was appropriate, that she had in fact targeted all the appropriate preschools, and that it made sense that she felt so distraught. She was merely mirroring the feelings of many other parents, like the mother of a four-year-old boy, Andrew, who described her reactions upon finding out about another four-year-old boy in her community who had a tutor to help him with math and reading: "This makes me nervous. If the other kids have tutors, will Andrew need one, too?"[2]

I agreed with Arielle's mother that yes, it would be better if we could stop all the pressure and children could just be the little children they're supposed to be. But I knew that it was going to be a big step to help her consider the next possibility of "jumping ship"—casting off her worries about whether she was doing enough and dropping her desperate attempts to keep up with her cohorts in assuring an optimal, high-achieving childhood for her daughter. From where she sat, she perceived the current that was sweeping her along as far stronger than both her and me, a current driven by the mass insecurities and generalized anxiety about work, family, politics, and economy in the culture at large. Despite her own good sense that it should be otherwise, she felt she could not afford to leave the quick-moving stream that carried both her and her daughter forward in the race toward adulthood. Even though she had an inkling that "It's crazy what we're doing," she experienced the situation as totally beyond her control. Instead, to affirm that her little daughter would be able to keep her head above water, she believed she needed to steer a course for her child through the best schools in town.

I knew my immediate reassurances were only a finger in the dike, and in no way solved the larger problem for this family. I also had a gnawing feeling that I had not gotten to the heart of the problem. Without better intervention, the combination of social pressures and this woman's own psychological makeup was leaving her at risk for "chronic parental anxiety syndrome," if there was such a clinical diagnosis. Her husband's passivity and lack of clarity on the issue of baby's achievement would only exacerbate the angst.

Arielle's parents left the consultation feeling they got what they came for, to be reassured that they had targeted the right schools. They were not interested in a follow-up appointment. Not able to take the next step with them, I did not feel successful in my consultation. Perhaps I had treaded too lightly, offering too much understanding and reassurance and not enough probing or confrontation. But that is not what they came for and I assessed, I now think wrongly so, that they would be resistant to anything but the answer to their question about preschool planning.

After they left, I sat thinking, "These people will surely be back in my office in the future, the next time they fear for their child's accomplishments and doubt their own efficacy in assuring success for her." Perhaps then there will be a second chance to entertain the notion of getting out of the rat race—when they are more open or when they have had more years of hand wringing. They could then begin to think about the possibility that their daughter's life would be just fine even if she did not go to the top-notch preschool and even if she did not have her pick of the best colleges later on. Maybe it would even be better, allowing her to follow her own path rather than the path of perfectibility carved out for her by others. Feeling guilty that I hadn't stepped in sooner, I thought how much more sane and happy these parents could feel if they could turn the tide on their anxious preoccupations and find the freedom simply to enjoy their very young child as she rolled along into toddlerhood.

The ideal solution to this family's predicament sounds a bit like, "If everyone would just put down their guns at the same time, there would be no more war." But no one wants to risk being the first to disarm. So parents fortify themselves with pushing and prodding and sending their children to every available school, class, lesson, training, or cultural experience aimed at bettering their future.

The anxiety about our children "making it" wipes out our common sense, even in the most sane of parents. This anxiety propels us to push and hurry our children so. There have always been neurotic and hand-wringing parents. But now the anxiety seems to have reached epidemic proportions and is highly focused on achievement markers in the children. The content of those markers may vary from family to family—one set of parents may be pushing their children toward mathematical wizardry, while another mother and father may want a well-rounded "Renaissance" child. But regardless of content of the markers, the aim is the same—shoot for the top.

Yet in psychological theory it is almost a truism that anxiety is the handmaiden to guilt or vice versa. Parents are not only anxious about their children's future. Their parental guilt slips in—they themselves have done hardly enough to be the "good enough parent" who instills a sturdy sense of self in their children, a task they take very seriously and take full responsibility for. So the guilt and anxiety feed off each other, and the pushing only gets more intense.

Parenting by guilt rears its mighty head to help create the ill-fitting image of "my toddler, the doctor." The overscheduling, overstimulating, and overpromoting of our children is both an expression of and an attempt to alleviate this guilt that dominates our parenting. At some deep level, we've gotten the cockeyed idea that all this pushing, which we mask as "encouragement" or "support," is the best way to make up for our lack of availability, our preoccupation with other things, our own stress levels, and our distress that we cannot offer to our children the same promise our parents offered to us, that the world will be their oyster. However, we can learn more fully how the guilt, anxiety, and concern with pushing our children to perfection come together to create an unsettling experience for both parent and child. With this understanding, we can remove ourselves from the entrapment of "my toddler, the doctor" and find new ways to help our children truly reach their fullest potential. Let us start with an investigation of what exactly this perfection that we are trying to instill is.

WHAT KIND OF PERFECTION ARE WE SHAPING?

Long ago, the perfect child was the one who was seen but not heard. If we go back to the 1920s, we can find a description of the ideal child as the child who "never cries unless actually stuck by a pin . . . who puts on such habits of politeness and neatness and cleanliness that adults are willing to be around him at least part of the day . . . who eats what is set before him . . . who sleeps and rests when put to bed for sleep and rest . . . who finally enters manhood so bulwarked with stable work and emotional habits that no adversity can quite overwhelm him."[3]

I don't think any of the parents we are talking about here would find cause to celebrate if they produced such a child. No, they would find that child repressed, depressed, unassertive, or uninspired. Instead, today's perfect child is content, competent, confident, communicative, and demonstrates *outstanding* skills in at least one if not several arenas of life. That's what parents want.

We get a window into the concept of the perfect child by listening to a father who thinks he does not have one. Anthony is a fifty-year-old father of a nine-year-old son, Jordan. Anthony and his wife have a close connection with another couple in the community who have a son, Brandon, who is also nine. In Anthony's eyes, Brandon can do no wrong, while his own son, Jordan, always falls short. Brandon plays the piano beautifully and practices religiously an hour a day. Anthony's son is still stuck on scales and practices only when coerced. Brandon loves to play baseball. Anthony's son would rather retreat to his room. Brandon is always outgoing and self-possessed. Jordan is a shrinking violet. Brandon is industrious; Jordan is lazy, just sits around like a sloth in a tree. Jordan's father completely overlooks Jordan's gentleness; his abilities to entertain himself; his interest in model trains, planes, and cars; and his inventiveness in creating his own musical instruments from tin cans and spoons. He does not see these as fostering success in the modern world. In Anthony's narrative, his friend's son, Brandon—industrious, accomplished, and confident—is perfect. His own son—inward, musing, and creative—is a loser.

Anthony is driven by the modern notion of success, which does not, in his mind, include a lyrical, introverted child. He can overlook rather than delight in Jordan's virtues because they don't fit the mold of either what he would want for a son or what he thinks a son must have to make it in the world. (I should also mention that Anthony is equally hard on himself, always falling short when he compares his own to others' accomplishments). Anthony is in need of a major "realignment" in which he openly reevaluates his notions of success for his child and recognizes how his anxiety-driven, negative attitude toward Jordan's accomplishments and potential is creating the very failure he fears, as he subtly (and not so subtly) undermines Jordan's self-confidence. That is the therapeutic work Anthony and I are engaged in now.

I can't emphasize enough how important it has been for Anthony to do this work, for children are only too well aware of failing the criteria of "perfect child." Madeline is a radiant, soulful, and intense seventeen-year-old. Madeline "crashed" at the beginning of her senior year in high school. She no longer wanted to hang out with her friends. She broke up with her boyfriend. She increasingly lost any interest in going to school. Madeline reported tearfully to her mother that there was nothing special about her, nothing that stood out about her. She was just a nobody. Her mother tried to reassure her, but to no avail. All Madeline could remember were her father's words, "Be a star." Madeline had just embarked on her college applications. College counselors commonly advise that admissions committees look for something unique and special about an applicant. Madeline couldn't find any such thing about herself. This same "nobody" was accepted by almost every college she applied to. But such success did not alleviate Madeline's angst that she was a failure, a far cry from a perfect child—a child who would be happy and successful because she was a shining star in something.

Happiness and success are the two key elements of the modern ideal of the perfect child. Success is defined here as accomplishment in academic and artistic pursuits, in interpersonal relationships, in physical performance, and in personal development. Parents no longer have to worry as their ancestors did that their children might not physically survive the onslaught of incurable infant diseases or community epidemics. This frees us to substitute success and happiness for survival as goals for our children. Finally we can strive for the life promoted in the original declaration of our forefathers—exercising our inalienable rights of life, liberty, and the pursuit of happiness. High achievement becomes the ticket to reaching those goals.

Yet all the while, new threats to survival lurk in the shadows. The threat is no longer infant disease, but instead drugs, violence, sexually transmitted disease, or harm to oneself. The reappearing threat to survival shadows the pursuit of success and happiness. The pursuit and the threat are continually playing against each other throughout our years of child rearing, beyond those original days after birth when our soaring parental narcissism was pierced. We strive for perfection; we dread destruction.

FROM WHENCE COMES PERFECTION?

Anthony, the father mentioned above, lamented that nine-year-old Jordan fell so short of perfect. It certainly sounded as though

Anthony felt he had been dealt a bad hand or ended up with a lemon of a child. But it was not so simple. As he and I explored the roots of his disappointments in Jordan, we barely scratched the surface and out came an outpouring of self-castigation. He berated himself mercilessly for his own failure to produce such perfection in his child. He ruthlessly compared himself to Brandon's father, whom he perceived as fathering perfectly, and saw himself as grossly negligent and inept in comparison. He was ornery, unathletic, overly critical, and interpersonally clumsy. In his inability to separate himself from his son, he perceived that if he had a damaged child, it was only because he, a damaged and damaging father, had created him. Conversely, if he was an inept parent, the inevitable outcome was a damaged child. It is the parent who determines the child's destiny.

Anthony may feel clear about his culpability, but the scientific community around him is not nearly as steadfast in its position on this issue. No consistent line of thinking prevails about what goes into the development of a particular child. Debate abounds concerning the question of nature versus nurture.

There are two major schemas of childhood. One is the child as a tabula rasa, an empty slate on which parents and culture put their stamp and create the child from scratch. John B. Watson, the early twentieth-century behavioral psychologist, is perhaps the most famous spokesperson for this stance, insisting that he could take any infant and turn him or her into anything he wanted—lawyer, artist, beggar, or thief.[4] B. F. Skinner followed in his footsteps, raising his own daughter in a Skinner box, a perfectly controlled environment.[5]

The alternative schema is the newborn as a preformed being. In this scenario, the child is like a plant waiting to unfold. The responsibility of the social environment is to provide the watering can. In the 1940s, child developmentalists such as Gessell and Ilg were great promoters of this maturational model.[6] The shape and ultimate size of the being is predetermined in the seed itself. Nature rather than nurture is believed to be the driving force in development. Parents, rather than shaping destiny, stand on the sidelines and watch the inevitable process. Acculturation can never transcend maturation. From this way of seeing human growth, the various stage theories of development have evolved, in which human beings progress from one stage to the next in universal, fixed, and automatic progression.

As with many aspects of contemporary American child rearing, the tabula rasa and maturational conceptions of children's development have been fused so that nature and nurture are seen as inseparable. The argument, then, is that the development of the human being is always an interweaving over time of a child's constitution and the influence of the environment in which he or she grows. A depressed mother can create an anxious baby, but a constitutionally unsoothable baby can also create a depressed mother. One cannot deconstruct heredity and environment, because they are always intertwined.

This reciprocal model of development, which stresses the child as an active agent in his or her own development and attributes a fluid and plastic nature to both the child and the environment as the girl or boy moves through childhood, is a very sound and measured approach to explaining the development of one human being from birth to maturity. But parents and professionals alike, attempting to make sense of their own daughters'/sons'/subjects' growth, seem incapable of holding onto this comprehensive map, which embraces both nature and nurture. Removed from the developmental psychology laboratory to the popular sensibilities about children and parents, the reciprocal model has devolved into a polarized juxtaposition of acculturation and constitution, rather than an interweaving of the two. We are dizzied by a quick-moving vacillation between the two poles of heredity and environment. We can read one article documenting conclusive scientific evidence that at least seventy-five percent of intelligence is fixed in the genes, only to turn the page and find another article attributing children's intellectual success solely to parents' willingness and availability to monitor their children's schoolwork. We are in a quandary as to what really creates perfection and what is the cause of failure.

In my own clinical work I find myself having to shift from one extreme to the other in offering consultation to parents concerning the development of their children. One couple comes in to tell me that their child is a tyrant, ruining their lives, because she *won't* go to bed, eat what her parents serve, allow her parents a moment's peace alone, or show consideration for anyone but herself. Their child, Jenelle, is just three. I work carefully with the parents to help them recognize that Jenelle was not born a despot. She is simply adapting to the environmental messages, expectations, and feeling states that had been communicated to her both consciously and unconsciously by Mom and Dad: that she was allowed to do whatever she wanted, that no one ever set limits for her, that no one ever let her cry, that no one had ever considered curbing her demanding behaviors. They, particularly the father, had grown very angry at their "spoiled" child, and felt increasingly punitive and negative toward her. Unconsciously, these angry feelings may have been defenses against their own guilt and sense of inefficacy, but at a conscious level Jenelle's parents were surely operating from the premise that Jenelle was just made that way and was sent down from somewhere to torture them. I had to remind them that *they* had created this problem in their own overly permissive child-rearing approach and they couldn't blame Jenelle for that. She didn't ask to become a spoiled child. Instead, they could use their anger toward Jenelle as a warning signal that something needed to change and that, in fact, there is hope for a change in Jenelle's comportment if they could change their treatment of her, setting limits and accepting that frustrating some of her wants would not damage Jenelle.

In the same week, I counseled a family about their five-year-old's behavior problems at school. Rashid had been born with a congenital disorder of unknown origin that was similar to autism but had no clear-cut diagnosis. He was hesitant to interact with other children and often approached people with unbridled aggression when what he really wanted to do was just make friends. The parents anguished about what they and, alternatively, the school were doing wrong. Here was a child who was gifted intellectually; why was he so inept socially? I had to reiterate several times that Rashid's peer problems stemmed from the neurological components of his disorder. Whereas the parents certainly could help facilitate better functioning in his areas of disability or dysfunction, they could not push his little brain or psyche to go faster than it was prepared to go in negotiating his social world, which was going to be a whole lot slower than in tackling intellectual tasks, which he did with alacrity. It was very hard for the parents to stay focused on the maturational component of their son's behavior. To do so would be to accept the disheartening conclusion that there was nothing *they* could do to make their child normal. In a culture that glorifies the quest for perfectibility, such a conclusion becomes especially devastating. Also, in their heart of hearts, they really believed that it was they who were responsible for the creation of Rashid's problems, not because they thought they had passed on their own genetic flaws, but because of their deeply ingrained belief in the child as a tabula rasa.

Once they began to alter their perception of both themselves and their child, the situation with Rashid changed dramatically. I asked them to think of Rashid as if he had been born hard of hearing. Instead, he had been born "hard of socializing." Just as we teach hearing-impaired children signing or lip reading and provide them with hearing aids, Rashid needed to be both taught and provided with aids to ensure better relationships with the social world, rather than simply being left to his own resources or being pushed to do things beyond his own capacities. We designed a program to help Rashid have more successful interactions with his peers. Both his parents and his school would need to push sometimes, but as facilitators, not as "shapers" totally in control of his destiny and success. Rashid's behavior began to show marked improvement, and his parents were now able to enjoy rather than agonize about their interactions with their child. His limitations no longer filled them with a sense of failure, but reminded them of the sad but at the same time reassuring reality that Rashid's deficits came from his own wiring and that they were doing all that they could to help him cope with his "hard of socializing" problem.

The last decade of the twentieth century has brought with it a renewed emphasis on the role of heredity and genetics in the interactive model of human development, a shift that ought to help parents like Rashid's. This trend involves seeing the child as a well-formed being from birth: "A new born child is not a formless bit of clay waiting to be shaped by parents or anybody else. . . . Genes aren't the sole ingredient of the personality soup, they are merely the well-seasoned stock. This message should be liberating for all parents—and children."[7] Maturation forms the base; acculturation fine tunes.

Identical twin studies have been key in demonstrating that certain personality traits are indeed inherited rather than socialized. Research at the University of Minnesota comparing identical and fraternal twins raised apart found a strong genetic component to certain aspects of personality, such as social potency, traditionalism, stress reaction, aggression, and harm avoidance. Identical twins, sharing the same genetic structure, showed the highest levels of consistency on these factors, despite growing up in very different environments.[8] Other research demonstrates that certain children have an innate resiliency that prepares them to face adversity without untoward psychological damage. Pertinent attributes include the ability to seek out substitute caretakers, special talents and interests, the ability to develop a rich fantasy life, and persistence and the capacity to "bounce back" after an assault on development.[9]

Calling on the reciprocal model of development, there has been an attempt in the child development field to underscore the role of the child in shaping the environment. We are asked to remember that parents don't only rear the child, children also rear the people who raise them.

This sends a signal to parents that they are not solely responsible for who their child is or how he or she comes out, but at the same time they do get to play their hand in nurturing and shaping their child's innate potential. With this map to guide him, a father of a three-year-old can report: "We appreciate Martin for who he is, without the guilty anxiety that every vagary of his personality results from flawed parenting that reflects our own unresolved childhood conflicts."[10]

But is this really a liberating message to parents? And do most parents ever even hear it? The soothing words that the child makes the parent as well as the parent making the child are soon lost in a social milieu that remains relentless in holding parents ultimately accountable for child outcomes.

One morning I turned on a local news station to pass the time on the drive to my office. Within fifteen minutes of air time, I learned that children's failing grades were a result of parents' lack of availability to monitor their children's homework and that parents were responsible for the growing rates of obesity among children because they failed to provide proper diet and exercise to their offspring. My own children are not fat and they do not have failing grades. Yet I was incensed by these conclusions. Ranting to no one in particular as I drove along, I asked, "What about the tremendous cuts in funding for schools? What about shamefully inadequate teacher salaries? What about fast food pushed on children both in school cafeterias and shopping malls? What about fast food as convenient and affordable meals for children whose parents have no time to cook or are forced to leave their children to fend for themselves at mealtime? What about parents who cannot afford healthy food for their children?"

I knew the answer to my questions. In this country, the parents will still take the rap, as when a reporter for *Time* magazine concludes her piece on rising mental illness among children and youth by stating, "As necessary and beneficial as [psychotherapy] treatment may be, it makes better sense to prevent emotional turmoil among youngsters by improving the environment they live in. Most important, parents must spend more time with sons and daughters and give them the attention and love they need. To do less will guarantee that even more children will be struggling for sanity."[11] Yes, children need more time with their parents. Parents are only too well aware of how little there is. But surely a society that does not take good care of its children should take some of the rap for the children's emotional ailments.

It is no wonder that so many people today are jumping on the bandwagon of diagnosing their children as having attention deficit disorder. It's not that they want to label and drug their sons and daughters. Attention deficit disorder, considered a neurological ailment, is at least a syndrome that parents are not blamed for, except inasmuch as they pass it on to the children through the genes or through brain trauma upon exiting the birth canal. But at least their parenting is not at fault.

Despite all the documented research, mental health professionals remain typically unmoved by reports of children's natural endowments or deficits—they are staunch environmentalists when it comes to child development and parenting. Beginning with the schizophrenogenic mother of the 1950s, all explanations of child suffering lead back to Mother. As one clinician expressed it, "I cannot remember ever working with a mother—wealthy, middle class, or poor—who did not have secret theories about how behaviors, or choices, or feelings of hers had deeply harmed her children."[12] The only way mother blaming has been altered, unfortunately, is by generously extending the accusations to fathers.

From a parent's point of view, the blame-the-parent syndrome directly replicates the experience of Alice when she enters the Queen's court in Wonderland. As if speaking of the authorities who stand in judgment of parents, Alice exclaims: "I don't think they play at all fairly, and they all quarrel so dreadfully one can't hear oneself speak—and they don't seem to have any rules in particular. At least if there are, nobody attends to them." As far as the Queen is concerned, there is indeed a structure: "Sentence first—verdict later."[13] When it comes to mothers and fathers, the sentence is clear: unrelenting guilt, anxiety, and exposure to the accusation that they repeatedly fail their children, with no social supports to help fix what is broken. The verdict is fairly consistent: Guilty—of damage to the child due to negligence, self-involvement, overinvolvement, incompetence, or ignorance.

If the parent is capable of damaging the child, logic dictates that the parent is also capable of perfecting the child. Like the mental health professionals, parents are barely affected by the notion of the child as a well-formed being who just needs good watering. In parents' eyes, there is no question where child perfection comes from: ourselves. We live in an era that does not accept submission to destiny. You can present us with all the research you want about a child's inherited fixedness, but we still believe we can transcend nature and can find the means to control and perfect our destiny.

Elaine and Don have a son, Peter, who is highly uncoordinated physically. Nobody knows why but he's been that way since infancy. Over the years, Don and Elaine have taken him to physical therapists, occupational therapists, sensory integration specialists, orthopedic doctors, and remedial physical education classes. Going from one thing to another, they have now exhausted every resource in the community, and Peter is still uncoordinated. But they keep going, because they believe there is a cure somewhere—if not today, tomorrow. And the professionals play their part in encouraging them to keep going.

It is laudable for Elaine and Don to give Peter the best shot possible in life by getting him all the services he needs to remediate his weaknesses. If they could stop there, it would be fine. The problem is that they keep going. Their transcendental fervor is translated into the never-ending search for perfectibility. It is not just them. We are all guilty of that.

• • •

THE CHILD AS PYGMALION

Parents, trying to shape perfection in their children, are also aware that the odds are not in their favor. A 1991 poll conducted by the *San Francisco Chronicle* reported that eighty-four percent of six hundred Bay Area residents responded that it was harder to raise children today than for their parents: "There's a bigger gap between what we think we should do and what we can realistically do. There are more demands outside the home, and there are higher expectations for what you should do to be a good parent inside the home."[14] The qualifications for "good enough parent" have risen dramatically. Simultaneously, the opportunities to meet these qualifications have plummeted radically.

But like Professor Higgins with Eliza Doolittle, parents are only too eager to engage in a hands-on marathon to mold their child into the most elegant, eloquent being he or she can be. We ignore the warnings, succinctly expressed by psychoanalyst Alice Miller: "As soon as the child is regarded as a possession for which one has a particular goal, as soon as one exerts control over him, his vital growth will be violently interrupted."[15] We protest that our child is not our possession, but rather our charge and that we do not wish to control but to offer our support, guidance, and encouragement. But where do we draw the line between helping and living through our child?

As one parent announced unabashedly in a consultation with a therapist: "It is very important to give our children the best middle-class life we can give them." That is why this parent is sending all three of his children to the most expensive private school in the area. When another parent found that her son had not been accepted to the nursery school of her choice because he was too far down on the waiting list, she wept and suffered sleepless anxiety: "I felt like Harvard had rejected me. I felt so irresponsible, and I tried to figure out where I had failed. It was crazy."[16]

This mother's misery might have been mitigated if she could have stopped and said to herself, "My pressure on myself to be the omnipotent parent who can shape a young superstar able to compete with the mightiest is not helping my son feel good about himself nor is it a realistic expectation of myself. The conditions in which we

must raise our children are indeed crazy when three-year-olds have to take entrance exams and there is not space for every child to have a stimulating and enjoyable preschool and day care experience. What will really be so terrible if he goes to a different kind of day care? What indeed are my other options for preschool? Is it really him or my investment in myself as a parent who has a child in such and such school that is at stake? If I were not worrying about his school rejection so much, what might I be doing instead that would be more beneficial for my son? Maybe he needs me to play with him rather than worry about him right now."

When the "This is crazy what I'm doing" bell goes off, the technique of posing such questions to ourselves can snap us out of our spiraling anxiety. Although it sounds rather mechanical or simplistic, I have found that, when integrated with psychological insight about our parenting by guilt and our chronic parental anxiety syndrome, it actually serves as effective "thought control." By engaging in an internal dialogue with ourselves and creating a new "antipushing" narrative, we shift not only our attitudes and feelings, but also our ensuing behavior with our children. Such a dialogue also infuses us with a sense of agency about what we *can* do to facilitate our children's happiness and success rather than leaving us stuck on what we have failed to do to enroll them in the best.

COME AND BUY PERFECTION

We will also have to resist pressures from the marketplace. The fast-growing industry of infant stimulation barrages us with high-priced paraphernalia that will stimulate our child's growth and development even before our child leaves the womb. An expectant mother is enticed to purchase a contraption that will gird her distended abdomen and deliver complex sonic patterns to her yet unborn baby, giving it the ultimate "headstart" in development, exciting the fetal nervous system and exercising the baby's brain. The item costs approximately 250 dollars. One mother reported that the sonic belt seemed to be a good way to give her child "as much of an opportunity as possible to see if it would stimulate her thought process."[17] Other pregnant mothers use home remedies,

holding speakers to their abdomen to stimulate their fetus's musical abilities.

The market peddles flash cards for nine-month-olds and educational videos for children well short of their first birthday.[18] Wimmer-Ferguson Child Products, which sells educational toys for babies, advertises their "Stim-Mobile": "an intelligent mobile, it promises to give you a more alert, more content, quieter baby." Their Double Feature, mirror on one side, seascape pattern on the other, offers "*double* the play value for babies and *double* the dollar value for parents." The advertising packet asserts: "Research indicates that infants given a visually enriched environment are less fussy and are more frequently quiet and attentive when awake than infants who are not given special stimulation. . . . Babies given these kinds of stimulation show sustained developmental advantages over infants in less stimulating environments."[19] The academic researchers agree. In 1996, Dr. Craig Ramey at the University of Alabama reported to the American Academy for the Advancement of Science that infant stimulation beginning as early as six weeks could increase babies' scores on intelligence tests by fifteen to thirty percent. This made front page news.[20]

Baby training packets sell, particularly to high-achieving parents with money to spare but little time to spend with their children. Lured by reports of two-year-old ice skating stars and preschool chess champions, a new sensibility prevails that children are capable of so many more things if we only give them the opportunity and the encouragement, beginning with twirling mobiles and high-priced, fancy mirrors. In this regard we can see the "miniature adult" end of the kinderdult in full regalia.

Parents also feel pressured that if they do not invest in these revolutionary advances in infant stimulation their child will be left behind, crippled in his or her chances to get into a good kindergarten and ultimately a good college. It is highly doubtful that parents actually have the time to use all these contraptions. But even if the educational toys never leave their boxes, they only reinforce the race to perfection, already in full gear by toddlerhood.

The market is only too happy to shape and reinforce the image of the new Super Baby: "Under the supervision of Super Moms and Super Dads, Super Baby has the latest gadgets, the best reading materials. Her crib is so filled with the most appropriate objects that there is hardly room left for Super Baby to sleep."[21] Super Baby's purchased infant education is only matched by the mother and father's parent education, the phenomenon of a generation of parents who school themselves with books and expert advice as they wend their way through child rearing. We would do better to keep our wallets in our pockets and rely far more on the old pots and pans and bits of string that are just plain fun. Our children will have plenty of time and opportunities to sharpen their intelligence.

PUSHY PARENTS, PERFORMING PROGENY

A thank you note comes to us from a colleague of my husband. We had sent his infant daughter a musical toy. The note reads, "My Dad says that's the best song to ski to in the whole world, I mean the one the train-music blaster you gave me plays, you know, 'This old man, this old man. . . . ' He says he used to sing it going over the moguls. That's crazy. I really like it. Maybe I'll be Mozart next year and play my own music. Come visit me. I'm crawling all over the place. It really helps to be able to get around. Love, Erica. My Mom and Dad send their love too." Clever and sweet, the underlying message does not escape us, and leaves a chill. Are these words the innocent reveries of a father steeped in expectable parental narcissism when soaring fantasies are understandable and acceptable? Or are they an expression of a father's undue expectations for professional prowess before little Erica has even left the crib?

In Manhattan, there is a program called French for Tots. One child, age three and a half, had already been a student in the program for a year and a half. Her mother wanted her to have the opportunity to be bilingual and had herself spent six years of her adolescence unsuccessfully trying to master the language. She also wanted her daughter, an urban child with no backyard, attic, or basement to play in, to be able to *do* something: "What was she going to do? Just sit around and play with her toys all day, seven days a week."[22] Not such a bad idea, for a two-year-old, but this mother had her focus elsewhere—on the intellectual achievement of her preschool-age daughter. By age five, she hoped to produce the linguist she herself had never become. This mother reveals the sensibility of a generation that believes that all play and no work a failure makes.

On July 4, 1988, *The New Yorker* published a cartoon of a baby in a play pen, with no toys, but with a computer plugged in for her perusal. Such children are now commonly referred to as "children in the fast lane." Showered with flash cards by age one, music programs by age two, and reading readiness by age three, the sensibility is that getting to the top is best and that growing equals learning equals achievement, period. A mother steps back and reflects: "We compress their time and pack it with play dates, lessons of all kinds and enriching experiences like camping and skiing. I can't help asking myself what worlds will they have left to conquer? We have introduced them in a few years to all the things we've grown to love or value in 30. My husband studied karate in college, I did tai chi in my 20's, but our son is an orange belt at 5."[23]

A father, a colleague of mine, sits across from me at lunch and explains that he has enrolled his four-year-old in a musical keyboard class. He has noticed that Alex's fine motor functioning, particularly his manual dexterity, is relatively weak. He wants to correct the deficit now, to give his child every chance to soar, to become a Mozart, like little Erica, if he so chooses. This father is earnest in his concern for his child, but it is as if his child has been transformed into a complicated machine studied microscopically by a doting father to make sure each of the separate mechanisms is perfectly gauged and calibrated. No thought was given to whether Alex would have *fun* at the keyboard lessons. That was irrelevant. The lessons will benefit him and his future. Enjoyment seems to have dropped out of the picture completely or at least has been overshadowed by accomplishment as the thing we owe to our children. And I don't see very many of our children thanking us.

I give you this litany of tales to document that middle-class American parents are caught in an endless web of achievement anxiety in trying to mold their children to perfection. But lest one thinks that excessive performance striving emanates solely from the parents, here is the story of a thirteen-year-old girl applying to a public alternative high school in San Francisco. A mother reports to me that she took her child to this school for her preacceptance interview and sat in while her daughter was being interviewed. The school interviewer asked this eighth grader what she planned to major in in *college.* Sharon, the daughter, stared blankly at the interviewer and imploringly searched her mother's face for a cue as to how to respond. Nancy, the mother, sat dumbfounded, her mouth agape. She was of no help to her daughter. The interviewer went on to inform Sharon that a great deal of attention was given in their high school program to *career* counseling. Nancy spent several hours after the interview reassuring her daughter that it was perfectly fine for Sharon's major focus right now to be getting along with friends, getting assignments done, and demanding girls' rights at her junior high. At thirteen, there was no need for her to know what she was going to be when she turned thirty. Had she the choice, Nancy would have withdrawn her daughter's application from this school. But as a single parent with limited income, her only other alternative was the local public high school that was understaffed and overpopulated. Ultimately, she took fate in her hands by moving to another community with a saner school system. Regretfully, pushing our progeny is not just the domain of parents. It has become institutionalized as our society's attitude toward our middle-class children.

Another thirteen-year-old met with the same problem as Sharon, in his extended family. His uncle kept asking him about colleges during a family visit to the East Coast. Did he want to go with his uncle to see Yale? Did he check out any colleges when he visited Boston? The boy replied, "No and no." The uncle, exasperated, pushed further, "Are you interested in Stanford then?" The boy finally blurted out, "I'm only going into the eighth grade."

Early adolescence, a time when Americans of a previous generation were free to either marvel or agonize over their budding breasts and changing voices, today becomes a time to declare a college major and set oneself on a career track. In a society concerned about the lack of direction among its youth and cognizant of the lack of opportunities actually awaiting our young upon their entrance into adulthood, social and public institutions spew out performance and achievement expectations as an insurance policy for the next generation. These pressures are also emblematic of the changing status of childhood, and our magnetic attraction to the miniature adult pole in those moments when we fear for our children's future. They also reveal adults' tendency to allow anxieties and pressures about their own accomplishments to spill over onto little people only a fraction of their age, who have their own developmental needs and predilections. This is a classic example of the blurring of boundaries between adulthood and childhood, which appears to benefit no one.

Even before high school entrance time, we see the meshing of parents' and social institutions' achievement pressures on children when we take a look at the kindergarten readiness movement that emerged in the 1980s. In the shifting educational arena, kindergartners were now expected to do what traditionally had been first grade fare—reading, writing, simple math. Desk work replaced block play. Some have argued that this upgrading was a function of so many children today attending preschool and having already gone through a "kindergarten program" of activities by the time of school entrance. But that does not explain why so many children were now being turned away from kindergarten programs at age five and told to come back when they were six and more "ready" for the kindergarten curriculum.

When I attended kindergarten in the early 1950s, you were "ready" if your fifth birthday came before a certain date in the fall of that year. It was an actuarial assessment. Now in many school systems across the nation, prospective kindergarten students are assessed, measured, and screened with a battery of tasks and tests. If the school system deems that they are not academically ready, the children are turned away until the next year and their parents are told by the educational authorities to "give your child the gift of an extra year of childhood."[24]

It is dubious that the educators' main intent has been to preserve childhood for today's young and provide them with a little extra. If that was their intent, they would keep kindergarten as it traditionally had been, a time for free play, exploration, and learning the ropes of school rules and routines. Instead, we witness the ill-thought-out shift in educational focus from play to "work," based on the new, singular emphasis on cognitive achievement. The shift is fueled by the pressure from both parents and educators alike to demonstrate that our children can do more and better earlier if we just give them the opportunities and the training. The roots of this achievement drive go back to the late 1950s. After the Soviets launched Sputnik, Americans felt compelled to compete, focusing much of their attention on the educational system and the Cold War rubric that "Anything they can do, we can do better."

By the 1990s, we are sobered by the research that suggests that kindergarten early readers become disillusioned and dispassionate students by age nine and that adult-stimulated early achievement in young children can result in anxious learners later. Children exposed to too much early stimulation may be candidates for stress, stomach aches, headaches, eating and sleeping problems, and plummeting self-esteem.[25] But, unfortunately, most parents are not exposed to this research, and even if we are, our worry about our children's achievement gets the best of us. So we continue to push. As we do so, we find ourselves trapped in our double vision of the kinderdult. We swing toward the "miniature adult" in our emphasis on children's "adult-like" thinking and performance traits in their formal rearing.

That kindergarten readiness is really a euphemism for our preoccupation with achievement is revealed in the number of parents who now *voluntarily* hold their children back a year before kindergarten entrance. Some parents do this to protect their children from undue academic pressure, which they recognize in the new upscale kindergarten programs that require entrance tests and interviews. They hear stories like the one from a mother who attended a kindergarten orientation program in which the teacher strongly advised the parents against putting too much stress on the children, only to discover that the same teacher then assigned homework to her little son on the very first day of school.[26] They want none of this for their own child.

But other parents have a different agenda: If they hold their child back a year it will ensure that he or she will perform better and soar to the top of the class. They have heard about the research demonstrating that six-year-old entering kindergartners far excel five-year-old entering kindergartners in grades and achievement tests throughout their schooling.[27] Of course, the parents' plan breaks down if every other child turns out to be just as old and prepared as theirs in the entering kindergarten class, but their dream is to see their advanced, well-sized six-year-old shining in a class of more immature, less developed five-year-olds. From kindergarten success will come the confidence for first-grade excellence, and from there an assurance of a Harvard acceptance. In either case—the parents who protect or the parents who push—the voluntary holding back of their kindergarten-age children is centered around the cult of success we've created for our children.

There is nothing magical about age five as the time to begin formal education. In many societies, children do not begin school until age seven, when it is believed that the child first reaches a developmental stage in which he or she will benefit from a formal instructional program. So what is the big deal about the shift from age five to age six as an average age of kindergarten entrance in our country? It reveals not an official shift in our age grading in the American educational system, but a strange contradiction: Our overemphasis on success and achievement becomes linked with a delay in our children's opportunity to enroll in school. Whereas a relaxed learning and play experience was assured to all five-year-olds of past generations, now children are turned away until age six and then faced with a grueling fast-paced kindergarten regime. With the school systems reinforcing parents' internalized achievement angst, is it any wonder that parents bite the bait so readily to push early learning, high achievement, and premature commitment? In the words of one mother, "Sometimes I feel that we've all entered a sweepstakes for the most accomplished person in the world in the year 2025, and that we've got to get ready *now*."[28]

UNDOING THE KNOT OF ANXIETY, GUILT, AND PUSHING

Two women I know are both gifted educators, well established in their fields and highly respected for their sensitivity to children's educational needs and their ability to focus on the "whole child." But when it comes to their own children, both these mothers have blind spots.

One has her children in two of the top private schools in the Bay Area, schools other children have to wait years to get in to, or never get accepted to at all. Yet she has only complaints about the schools. One of her children is bored in math. The other child suffers from a school curriculum that the mother perceives as dry and unbalanced. Neither she nor her husband can accept either of the schools as "good enough." They can only worry, incessantly, that their two children are not getting what they need.

The other woman is filling out kindergarten applications for her daughter: There are three hundred applicants for approximately ten spaces in her first-choice school. She obsesses with me about filling out the application. She's thinking of putting down "tomboy" as one of the adjectives to describe Emily on the application, but wonders whether that will increase Emily's chances or work against her as a candidate. She also wants the school to recognize, as she does, what a special child Emily is.

It is hard to break through these women's agonizing. In the moment the fretting seems intractable. If these two colleagues had been in my consulting room, I would have empathized with their frenzied state and then asked them to step back and take a look at what might be propelling their agitation. I would be operating under the assumption, until proved otherwise, that we are all able to work toward new and better perspectives on what we are doing. I would be focusing particularly on the following questions: Who are you doing this for—yourself or your child? If you communicate to them how anxious you are about their not getting the perfect education or not being recognized for being as special as they are, will that really help them negotiate in a world that is, indeed, far from perfect? Then I would ask, "We all want to do everything we can to ensure the best for our children, but really, what is the 'best'?" Some parents may feel angry and misunderstood when these questions are posed, but my intent is not to pressure, but to take the heat off of parents—to open up the possibility of breathing a little easier and worrying a little less. It often involves communicating to parents, both at a superficial and deep level, that (1) they have already done more than their share, now it is time to step back; and (2) it will not be the end of the world if the outcome is less than perfect. In fact, it may even be better for their children in developing resiliency and frustration tolerance.

A father calls me in distress because his son has just received notice that he did not get into any of the high schools of his choice. He and his wife had prepared their child for high school entrance from the time he was two. He had every lesson imaginable, along with ones that we could hardly conceive of. He had private tutors attend his school to offer him individualized enrichment programs. He had been promoted since his early years as a "very special child," which everyone around him both accepted and reinforced as he grew. Indeed, he was a child of many talents, but so are many other children. Clearly, the schools to which he had applied thought likewise. Soon after the father's distressed call, I also had opportunity to speak with the mother. In addition to the disappointment and shock about her son's rejections from the schools, she was consumed with guilt that perhaps she and her husband had not done enough to ensure his entrance—review his applications with him, monitor his preparation for entrance tests more carefully, push him a little harder. Her husband had remembered his own disappointments and failures from childhood, and felt guilty that he had been unable to shield his son from the same. The outcome: They began to push and promote their son even harder.

If they had not been blinded by their guilt and anxiety and could have stopped to consider not that their child was rejected, but that their child was *telling* them something very important in not getting accepted, a better end might have culminated for parents *and* child. He indeed didn't put much effort into his applications because he was fed up with all the pressure and longed for a slower pace that better fit his temperament. Perhaps he would be better off at the local high school where he would not be among the company of other "perfect" children and could determine his own pace. Perhaps he was not as invested as his parents were in being high achieving. Perhaps he did not want to face the upper-middle-class blackboard jungle, where As and awards substitute for switchblades and razors. Perhaps his parents might have recognized that they have been doing too much of one thing, pushing him to be the best, at the expense of doing too little of another, listening to him and what he wants for himself.

These parents, rather than feeling passive and victimized, mobilized all their forces to reverse, successfully, the schools' original rejections. But I would entertain an alternative solution: to think about what this situation was telling them about a possible shift in direction to take with their son and an alternative, potentially positive path their son might be carving for himself in not getting into the top high schools.

I can hear the objection loud and clear: "Our son can get lazy and really needs our help in pushing himself harder. It is just a matter of keeping options open. If we don't help him in this way, we shut out opportunities for him later." Of course we want to help our children develop to the fullest of their potential and have as many opportunities as possible available to them. Our biggest struggle, in the context of parenting toward perfection, is to be able to draw the line between helpful helping and overzealous pushing. It is a particularly hard delineation because the line between the two is often so blurred.

My husband and I were always grappling with what, to us, felt like a fine line between helping and pushing. To this day, my grown children still roll their eyes when they hear "keeping your options open." Yet we still hold firm to this as a measuring rod that helped us determine when to step in and "help" and when to catch ourselves "pushing" for our benefit rather than theirs. But we first had to ask ourselves, "What are our expectations for our children? Are they realistic?"

Research and experience both inform us that setting higher expectations for people in fact produces higher performance. But only within certain limits and often with potential fallout. For example, a mother told me of setting a standard of a B+ average for her son in order for him to be able to drive. Unfortunately, this child was truly not a B+ student, given his present academic abilities and the standards of the school he attended, where Cs were considered quite respectable grades. He didn't make the goal. It would have been better to set a more realistic standard for him and then help him reach that goal rather than to push him beyond his present capabilities, and then confront him with the failure to earn driving privileges. As for potential fallout, it is only too evident in the apathy and withdrawal from learning that surfaces in nine- and ten-year-old children who have been pushed into early reading and academic performance.

Returning to my own family struggles about helping versus pushing, once my husband and I determined whether our expectations were realistic, we then had to ask, is this only what *we* want or is it what our children want (or need), too? Over the years we learned that sometimes we simply have to say, "Well, it's good for them, like brushing teeth, even if they don't want to." But other times we have to listen very carefully when they become recalcitrant (e.g., consistently "forgetting" to play that violin) or when "helping" them unravels into power struggles, temper tantrums, or just bad times. Then we are either not helping in the right way or we may be unnecessarily pushing rather than stepping back and letting them struggle through something themselves. To "help" may be to give them the opportunity to find their own way to the finish line; to "push" may be to get overinvolved and overbearing—too much "in their face."

How we draw the lines between helping and pushing will certainly vary from one child to another, from one situation to another, and even from one parent's personality to another's. But no matter what the circumstances, checking ourselves for undue pushing is a good corrective to help us avoid seeing our children as Pygmalions that can be molded to perfection. It is better to see them as twigs that can only be bent so far and as children, who, no matter how gifted, will have to face an imperfect world with both their strengths and their weaknesses. Then we can confront our chronic parental anxiety more effectively and make room for our child, the child—rather than our toddler, the doctor.

It is easy for us as outside experts to counsel parents that it is not in their child's best interest to be pushed so much. But when you are operating from the inside, as a parent, both your own internal guidelines and the external social practices leave you bereft of any helpful clues to answer successfully the question, "Who am I doing this for, me or you?" As long as we assume that parents put pressure on their children solely because of their own narcissism, we will miss the totality and complexity of their internal experience. Narcissism and perfectionism are certainly alive and well. But if we can also keep in mind that mothers and fathers of this generation do not trust the wisdom of their own parental judgment, we can empathize with or at least more fully understand their driven behavior regarding their children's accomplishments. In a social system where the tabula rasa concept of childhood is nearly intractable, where parents are held ultimately responsible for both their children's feats and foibles, and where our "postmodern" culture has all but eliminated social guidelines for parenting by offering a pastiche of often contradictory child-rearing advice and information, the pressure to push in the age

. . .

of human perfectibility weighs heavy on parents who were raised to "have it all" and expect the same for their children.

The way out is a thorny path, but one well worth taking. It involves having the courage to drop out of the rat race as we differentiate between helping and pushing and use not just our children's successes, but also their failures, to inform us as to who they are and what they are telling us about where they want to go.

CHAPTER SIX

· · · · · ·

Pampering Our Children toward Success

The drive for autonomy can be strengthened by giving children the opportunity to practice new skills until they are mastered. At the same time, as children grow older, their urge to learn and mature can be impaired if their parents are constantly directing and dominating them necessarily, filling every waking minute with dictated activities.

—BENJAMIN SPOCK[1]

In pushing their children, parents create the new phenomenon, "my toddler, the doctor"—a mere little child capable of doing great things. Only two and he can already read beginning flash cards. Four and already a violin player, following in Mozart's footsteps. If it was just that parents pushed their children too hard, we could stop the story here. Many do. We could write a postscript reminding parents they have toddlers, not doctors, and our job would be done.

Regrettably, the tale is not so simple. When it comes to their children's achievements, parents do not just push. They also make the mistake of pumping their children up and setting the stage for children thinking that everything they do is a grand feat or a miracle. Parents want their children to feel good about themselves. To this end, they occasionally actually take over and do things for the children; they overvalue all of their children's accomplishments, no matter how large or small, while simultaneously undervaluing the children's capability or need to do things on their own. In this sense mothers and fathers are hardly pushing, but instead are pampering their children toward success.

The cult of success struts in full regalia. But if we zoom in on parents' interactions with their children, we discover that children are receiving a very mixed message. Parents run back and forth between pushing and pampering in the quest for star-studded children. It is this overlooked pampering that I want to address in the context of the new "my toddler, the doctor."

A daughter has an algebra exam. Her mother stays up all night with her studying. A father teaches his three-year-old to tie his shoes. The son's new feat is celebrated with a party and balloons. Parents become overinvolved and overzealous about their children's accomplishments. They are hell bent on building their child's self-esteem. The result: They coach and coddle at the same time. That is what is so dangerous about the present epidemic of chronic parental anxiety in the quest for perfectibility. Only by factoring parents' "preening for success" into the equation of parents' achievement anxiety can we see the full craziness of "my toddler, the doctor." With that insight, we can take the means to correct the craziness so that we are truly helping our children move forward rather than impeding their blossoming in life.

LET'S GIVE A BIG HAND TO THE CHILDREN

The first thing we need to comprehend is that a very odd phenomenon has evolved in American child rearing, which both feeds into and reflects our present plight of overblowing our children's accomplishments. I am referring to the new "self-esteem" movement that has grown so popular in American culture and has strongly infused our daily practices with our children: We are intent on having a people who feel good about themselves and what they do with their lives.

The application of the new "self-esteem" ethic runs the gamut from large corporations to kindergarten classrooms. Managers learn about ego-boosting among their staff. Teachers learn about positive reinforcement schedules. The focus is on feeling positive and reaching one's full potential in a supportive environment. We want to eliminate any negative feelings that people might have about their level of achievement, no matter what the achievement actually is. The goal is self-confidence and a good sense of self, without which, it is believed, success is impeded.

When we apply this ethic to children, it takes on a particular saliency to which we should give some careful thought. It appears that both parents and the country at large sing words to our children that are wildly discordant from the music to which they are sung. Regarding both ourselves and our children, we acknowledge the sense of cut-throat competition that ensues when striving to make it to the top of the pyramid amidst shrinking opportunities. Yet we speak words saying that competitive social and work relations are destructive and unproductive and should be replaced by a more "user-friendly" collaborative and cooperative spirit. So we focus on words and actions that lend themselves to support and ego boosting, all while the music of the rat race plays on.

In our relationships with children, the self-esteem ethic translates into every child receiving a star on the spelling test, not just the ones who scored 100%. "E for effort" and accolades for just trying are the new norms for positive reinforcement. A trophy is no longer reserved for the best player, but is awarded to every member of the team, just for being a teammate. Self-esteem building begins at the earliest ages with huge applause and cheers of appreciation for each step taken or every new word spoken. A toddler cleans her plate completely and the whole table bursts into song. You can buy a potty that plays "God Bless America" each time a child has a successful bowel movement.

From a child's point of view, every routine accomplishment becomes a major event for which the band plays. Children may not be given anything important to do, but every unimportant event becomes the equivalent of climbing Mount Everest. By the time a child reaches adolescence, his or her room can look like a trophies museum—a medal for attending camp, a certificate for *joining* a scouts program, a ribbon just for entering a painting in the school arts competition. The happy face stickers, stars, and large applause are primarily just for *being* rather than an acknowledgment of one's real accomplishments.

The purpose of the self-esteem movement is to shower children with praise in order to build their self-confidence and allow them to experience success. However, the program will be effective in bolstering confidence only if the child does not recognize it as a sham. My observation is that many children do, leaving them bereft of the ability to differentiate for themselves between what is a real accomplishment and what is not. And when children *don't* see it as a sham, they are at risk for thinking they are much better than they are, the recipient of award after award for excellence. The self-esteem program also prevents children from learning that there may always be people who are better at something than you are and that's okay— your job is to try hard but also enjoy yourself, and someday you will get a trophy or recognition for the thing you *are* good at.

In a study conducted at the University of Michigan, Dr. Harold Stevenson found that American children rank far ahead of students in Japan, Taiwan, and China in self-confidence about their abilities in math. It is nice to know we have infused our children with such a positive sense of self. Unfortunately, this is marred by the fact that American students are far behind in their actual performance in math when compared to these other groups.[2]

Marilyn brought her nine-year-old daughter, Tiffany, for her therapy session. When I came to greet them in the waiting room, Marilyn eagerly pushed a piece of paper into Tiffany's hands, encouraging her to bring it in to show me. Tiffany reluctantly took the paper and slithered into my office. I asked her gently if she wanted to show me the paper. Her reply, "Not really." I asked her if she was upset with her mother for pushing her to bring it in. Her flat reply, "Not really." I said I guessed it was a certificate for something she had done and that she wasn't really enthused about telling me, and that we could just leave it at that. But then she decided she wanted to talk about it. It was a certificate of merit for her gymnastics class. Everyone got one for something special they had done. She got hers for her pretzel ties with her legs. But she said she was confused because everyone in the class could do pretzel ties with their legs. I asked her what she herself felt were her best accomplishments in gymnastics, the things she was most proud of. She said she had no idea.

As the conversation continued, Tiffany looked increasingly enervated and depleted. She actually loved gymnastics and had spent the last months enthusiastically demonstrating to me the new things she had learned. My own impression was that she was indeed very talented in gymnastics and was quite motivated to continue taking classes and improving her skills. In her case the delivery of accolades had not *inflated,* but, indeed, had *deflated* her sense of her own accomplishments.

I thought about the gymnastics teacher who probably wanted to help every child feel good about his or her progress and hoped through her certificate program to avoid a competitive and "graded" program for the children. And I thought about how enthusiastic Marilyn had been about her daughter's award. The problem was that the little recipient, Tiffany, wasn't.

In my next parent session with Marilyn and her husband, Donald, I reported to them my impressions of Tiffany's deflation rather than elation around her certificate. I questioned whether the teacher's award system was working for the children, or at least for their child. I remembered my own daughter's merit system of earning medals for a certain level of skill in her gymnastics program many years ago, before the self-esteem movement had taken off in this country. When the children reached a certain skill level, they got their next medal—a little like Red Cross swim cards. My daughter, excited about her accomplishments, still has her medals hanging on her wall. I shared this memory with the parents.

Marilyn and Donald had never thought about it that way, and in fact they, too, were following in the gymnastics teacher's path by giving Tiffany a weekly reward for every new trick she had learned in gymnastics, whether she had mastered it or not. At first they objected to my invitation to reconsider their and the teacher's reward system, protesting that they did not want to reinforce competition and bad feeling in Tiffany. But then I pointed out that their goal was not being met with their present "self-esteem" system, at least regarding bad feelings. They chewed on this for awhile, and then went home to discuss the gymnastics award system with Tiffany. Tiffany simply repeated to them what she had told me. On my recommendation, they and Tiffany talked to the gymnastics teacher together, who was a very kind and sympathetic teacher. Although she held fast to her noncompetitive award system, she made a point of having conferences with Tiffany periodically about her unique and particular strengths as a young gymnast and also the skills she had yet to work on and improve.

There also was some work to be done at home. As a real move toward bolstering her self-confidence, I thought that Tiffany was a good candidate for my "basket of goods, basket of not-as-goods" approach. This would involve Marilyn and Donald asking Tiffany to think about two baskets, one the "good" basket and one the "not-as-good" basket. Then she could sort out what she thought she would like to put in her good basket and what she would like to put in her not-as-good basket regarding her gymnastics accomplishments. This would allow her to see that there really were some things she felt she did well, even if she thought the certificates were meaningless. It would also help her assess for herself the things she would like to continue working on. At first, this might be very hard for her if she was really confused about her own accomplishments. But Marilyn and Donald could help her by sitting with her and doing their own two baskets for Tiffany, modeling for her their honest assessment of her successes and accomplishments. To make it less threatening for Tiffany, they could also do one for themselves, so Tiffany could see that not just little children but grown adults have things they do well and things they do not as well—it's just part of being a person. In that way Marilyn and Donald, too, would get some training in sorting out real accomplishments from false glory.

Donald and Marilyn reported in their next session that Tiffany was delighted to do "the basket thing," as she called it, and even insisted that they take two baskets and put them in a special place so the whole family could play basket of goods, basket of not-as-goods for all kinds of things. She particularly found great glee in assessing her parents' accomplishments (and shortcomings), which allowed her to lighten up about her own. Ironically, rather than engendering a more competitive spirit, Tiffany was now able to get genuine thrill from her own achievements and abilities and generously extend that feeling to other people and theirs.

What Marilyn and Donald learned is that we do no service to our children when, in our manic preoccupation with success and self-esteem, we inflate their egos through feedback that each tiny step forward or attempt to do *anything* is a monumental feat, worthy of a Congressional Medal of Honor and a major celebration. It more likely leads to deflation (or unrealistic inflation) rather than elation and would best be substituted with meritorious awards or none at all, simply accepting the moves forward without all the hoop-la.

Eliminating the overzealous clapping can also reduce the risks of deifying our children through the overvaluation of their childhood accomplishments. When we err in the direction of deification, we create individuals who think they are better than they are and feel good about a self that really can't do as many things as they think, which was never our intent. Although I proposed in the last chapter that the boy who got rejected from all the prestigious high schools may have been sending a message to his parents, there also may have been a message sent back to him that was the opposite of ego-boosting. Having been brought up to be a "very special person," at least in his parents' eyes, what a surprise to find out that all these schools did not also think so. Even if he wanted out of the academic blackboard jungle, he would nonetheless be at risk for an assault on his self-esteem and for the burgeoning of self-doubt as he faced the schools' rejections.

Joan and Jim had a child, Jason, who had studied the trombone since he was six. They encouraged his playing and had him perform at every family party, with great fanfare and applause. They referred to him as their little musical genius. He got to junior high and tried out for the community youth jazz band. The little musical genius had a lot of competition, and he didn't make it. His rejection letter came in the mail while he was at school. His parents hid it. Joan and Jim called me in a panic. Surely there must be some mistake. The band director had encouraged Jason to apply. Jason would be crushed when he found out he was not accepted. They were going to call the director right away to intervene on Jason's behalf. I explored with them the strong intensity of their reaction and how this might affect Jason. Were they really feeling for Jason or for themselves? I wondered whether it would actually be the end of the world if Jason didn't participate in the band. Perhaps, rather than lobbying behind the scenes for Jason's acceptance, Joan and Jim would do better to help Jason work through the inevitable disappointments that come with not being accepted, even when we are quite good at something. The harsh reality is that there may have been someone that was just a little better, and that he should try again next time there is an audition, because he is still a good trombone player. I don't know how effective this intervention was in cutting their anxiety, but I do think it allowed Joan and Jim to step back before acting. From a distance, they could recognize how their overzealous clamoring and clapping for Jason's success was only creating an anxious child unable to tolerate frustration and overly sensitized to his parents' own anxieties about his accomplishments. This stopped them from jumping in too fast to fix it for him. They pulled themselves together, gritted their teeth, and simply handed Jason the rejection letter. They discovered that Jason didn't take it as hard as they expected, and certainly not as hard as they had.

If we don't at least tone down the cheerleading for the children, they may come to expect a round of applause and shower of praise for every small act, which thwarts any opportunity to experience the positive effects of their accomplishments just for the intrinsic value and based only on their own internal feedback. The children also miss out on the opportunity to receive low-key but serious recognition when they truly have done something important for which they should be proud, and to manage their feelings when such recognition is not forthcoming. These missed opportunities rob children of the critical underpinnings of ultimate independence and accurate self-concept.

We parents have wandered off track in thinking that if our children *think* they are the best, they, in fact, *will* be the best. We think we can spoon-feed their self-confidence by indulging them with accolades and praise. We become fairy godparents who shield our children from any bad feeling and wave our magic wands filled with stickers and stars so that as in the fairy tale, our sons and daughters can believe that anything they touch will turn to gold.

But we never lose sight of the fact that it is gold that we want for them. We want them to feel good, but we also want them to make it in the world—to go right to the top. This dynamic drives us into the entanglements of pushing our children forward, and then stepping in to do everything for them to ensure their fame.

THE DISAPPEARANCE OF PLAY

As we preen our children for success and self-confidence, we get totally engrossed in applauding one major attribute—our children's cognitive precocity. The child who reads faster, does algebra sooner, and reaches Piaget's formal stage of thinking earlier becomes the epitome of the successful, self-confident child. Even the little songs that children sing are no longer just for the joy of it—they have an ulterior motive of demonstrating a child's brilliance and musical abilities.

Childhood may certainly not have disappeared, but, as a result of parents' desire for their children's success, one of its most critical centerposts, play, may well be on its way out. Jean Fitzpatrick, in *The Superbaby Syndrome,* eloquently states the problem: "By the 1960s, many parents were taking Maria Montessori's slogan 'Play is a child's work' as an invitation to switch their kids from hide-and-seek to hard labor."[3]

In the blurring of boundaries between childhood and adulthood, adults, accustomed to the work ethic of productivity, deadlines, schedules, and pay bonuses, now apply these same criteria to the world of children. In the context of rushed and harried family life, neighborhoods no longer safe for unsupervised play, and playmates spread all over the urban or suburban map, the scheduled "play date" has taken the place of spontaneous fun. Gone is the opportunity for hanging out on the sidewalks playing children's games and exploring the environment or just spending time in one's room. Parents' overscheduled lives are equally matched by the over-scheduled days orchestrated for their children. We used to think that children got into emotional trouble because they had too much free time on their hands. Now they are more likely to be at emotional risk because they have *no* time.

Not just children, but their parents as well suffer from the diminution of play in daily life. Americans work incredibly long hours with minimal vacation time. Parents trying to juggle paid work and family obligations repeatedly lament how time for themselves, leisure time, has disappeared. No opportunity exists to contemplate, or just do nothing.

Children get swept up in the mania of making every minute count. A mother describes to me her daughter's little friend, age six, a child from an overachieving family who have enrolled her in every activity imaginable. Just out of curiosity the mother asked her daughter's friend, "Do you play Barbie?" The little girl responded emphatically, "Oh no, I'm much too busy to play Barbie."[4]

• • •

We value happiness tremendously as a goal for our children, but we have lost sight of the ingredients that go into that happiness. Despite wide variations in race, ethnicity, and national character, there is such a thing as a universal "essential childhood." The essential child feels well, plays well, works well, eats well, thinks well, copes well, enjoys well, and expects well.[5] Unfortunately, there is a glaring omission of the second feature, "plays well," in the shifting American child-rearing practices.

First, let us establish what we mean when we speak of "play." It is more than a hopscotch game or marble game or "Let's pretend that. . . ." These are the activities children manifest when we give them the space and permission to explore their bodies, their environment, their thoughts, their feelings, and their imagination. But play as a psychological experience and a contribution to development is a much deeper phenomenon.

Play sets the stage for creativity in life. Creativity involves a coloring of our attitude toward the world so that we do not just respond to things literally as we see them but also inject subjective meaning, coming from our own imagination, into the experience. Play starts when we're babies and interact with our parents, creating a psychological space where we have a new experience of an aspect of life that is neither "inside me" nor "outside me," but resides somewhere in the middle.

The perfect early example of this is the teddy bear or favorite blanket. The baby attaches special meaning to the object, as a substitute for the comfort of a parent. If the baby were to be confronted, the baby would know full well that, after all, the blanket is really just a piece of cloth. But the baby is also quite clear that the blanket is far more than just a piece of cloth. The parent soon learns this, too, gleaned from the baby's poignant cries the first time the object is forgotten on a long family outing. This "transitional object" is a special possession that provides comfort and sustenance like no other inanimate object can. And nobody but the infant him- or herself can endow the object with such meaning. It belongs to the baby's arena of play.

For the growing child, play is a creative experience. It takes up space and it takes up time. It is intensely real for the child. The child gets to act in the world in a special and powerful way—taking things from everyday life and making them have special, personal meaning for the child. A child picks up a block of wood and transforms it into a truck just by going, "V-r-o-o-m, v-r-o-o-m, v-r-o-o-m." To any outside observer, the block is just a piece of wood. But to that child this object has been temporarily infused with imaginary wheels, windshield wipers, and racing engine. An hour later, this same child may cavalierly dump the fancy vehicle as just another piece of wood, but for the time being it is a sacred object.

Play, so defined, is universal and facilitates growth and therefore health. It is natural, if not obstructed, and later allows us to relate in full and meaningful ways to the people around us, contribute to the culture in which we live, express our inner selves, and have a sturdy sense of ourselves as subjects who can act on the world. It also allows us to find respite from the demands of daily life, finding relaxation through reverie, dreams, whimsy, and creative endeavors. Without it, we are left with rigid conformity and compliance to external demands, with no sense of a rich, flexible, inner existence that makes life worth living rather than a futile exercise. We see this all the time in the Type A workaholic who knows only how to put in twelve hours at the office, come home to make work calls, and then wake up the next morning to start the same routine all over again. And all the time, this person complains about feeling over-worked and empty. We see it in the fourteen-year-old anorexic who only knows how to get straight As, worry about getting straight As, and control her life through controlling her calories.

Ironically, in trying desperately to facilitate our children's fame by assigning a star for every feat, we may be inadvertently thwarting the very thing we are striving for—our children's growth, creativity, and health. The alarm has been sounded that American children today are squelched in their opportunities for play. With the great emphasis put on the early acquisition of formal learning skills and an award for every accomplishment, free play and fantasy have dropped in value and are only secondarily encouraged in children. Ignoring the need for children to ruminate, contemplate, and just do "nothing," we are instead obsessed with cheering them on and providing them with greater and greater opportunities to forge ahead in their cognitive development. For example, Fisher-Price reports that toys for five- to six-year-olds are now routinely bought for three- and four-year-olds.[6] I am also reminded of a colleague who confided in me that she became very distressed when her daughter would engage in outrageous dress-up games, and wished her daughter would play Monopoly instead and sharpen her mind. For this, the child would receive applause. And just last week, I opened the local newspaper to find a cartoon of a mother holding up a card from the box of "Smart Baby Flash Cards" and reading a letter from her baby: "After much introspection and consideration, I have concluded that I have reached a temporary intellectual saturation point. I am therefore temporarily requesting a brief sabbatical from the flash cards. Respectfully, The Baby."[7]

Productivity and excellence overshadow whimsy, fantasy, and emotional exploratory experiences as good outcomes for children. We would all agree that we want our children to be creative, but we have lost sight of how they might get there. Sometimes, children just want to be, they do not want to be cheered on, they do not want to be taken from one lesson to another to enhance their growth and development. Left from time to time to their own resources for play, they will indeed accelerate forward without the so-called benefit of the most accelerated and enriched learning experiences at our disposal and without a star for every accomplishment. All we need to do is give them the time and the space to play.

Increasingly in my clinical practice I meet up with children who lack the capacity to play. I am specifically reminded of a ten-year-old boy who came to see me for anxiety and behavior problems stemming from his parents' divorce six years earlier and the chronic tension in their relationship. Jonathan was a compellingly handsome child, well dressed, poised, and poignantly sad in his demeanor. He was very compliant in our first evaluation session. He drew the pictures I asked him to draw, responded to the questions I asked him to answer, told stories to picture cards that I showed to him, just as directed. Not once did he explore the playroom on his own. At the end of our session, he solemnly rose, shook my hand, and said, "Thank you very much, Dr. Ehrensaft. I so enjoyed meeting you. And I'm looking forward so much to going to the opera with my mother this Saturday." I stood somewhat dumbfounded as he sailed out of the office. I did not know whether this child had lost the capacity to play or never had it in the first place.

But his emotional constriction, his sadness, and his lack of vitality were palpable in the room.

Several months later, well into the therapy, Jonathan was able, in the playroom, to revisit the time in his life when his parents separated. No more opera and "Thank you, Dr. Ehrensaft" for this child. He chased me around the room in a pseudobaseball game in which tagging me out involved trying to bite me on the leg. All kinds of unlikely office accouterments and stuffed animals became bases. Guttural and animal noises abounded. He squealed in glee. Jonathan had developed the capacity to play.

Jonathan's parents had meant him no harm. They are part of the larger culture that advocates lessons, training, and structured activities for children. They thought he would feel good about himself if they gave him every cultural opportunity available and stretched his horizons as far as they would go. And ultimately, all he wanted was to curl up in his room, daydream, and play with a treasured toy rhinoceros that very much served as a "transitional object" for him, representing the parent he was missing.

Through our work together, Jonathan's parents discovered that they had other options. It was not just my therapeutic relationship with Jonathan, but also his parents' psychological changes that accounted for his developed capacity to play. In essence, it was a matter of a value shift. I told them point blank that Jonathan was suffering from an "adultomorphic" syndrome. He had fashioned himself as a little adult but that was just a false front, to himself and to others. He suffered from emotional constriction and general malaise as a result of it. Jonathan's parents were both taken aback, and it showed immediately on their faces. His father blurted out, "That's the last thing we want for Jonathan. We want him to be free to be him, not trying to be us." His mother wasn't so sure, she rather liked her precocious, sophisticated young son, and was hesitant to give that up. But she did share the following: "You know, I do think that both of us [she and her ex-husband] are guilty of extending our anxieties about our own work success onto Jonathan, and then we make him work as hard as we work and only applaud him for that." In our next session, I asked each of them to be a translator, to try to decipher the meaning of Jonathan's messages when he would (1) retreat to his room in defiance or (2) put on the false front (overly compliant, saccharine sweet) that was now becoming as obvious to them as it was to me. Through dialogue with each other and with me they got it. There were two clear messages: Lay off and let me be. Let me just be a kid.

This was truly a situation where insight led to dramatic behavioral change. Jonathan's mother stopped taking him to the opera. Both parents cut down on his extracurricular activities. They got rid of all the star charts. They came to recognize that doing nothing was doing something. The results were as palpable as his original emotional constriction, sadness, and lack of vitality. Jonathan became more relaxed, whimsical, and light spirited. He was happy. Several years later, his mother contacted me to let me know that he had gotten into a first-rate college, a testimonial to the fact that play and just "doing nothing" enhanced rather than impeded high achievement and academic success.

Parents, in attempting to ensure success and self-confidence, may instead induce in their children a conformity and adaptation to the world around them, with no room for exploration and originality. This, in turn, may produce a child who feels no sense of productivity and instead becomes dependent, inactive, unforthcoming, and unconstructive, not to mention uncreative. There is no genuine feeling of success on the child's part, and the child grows to feel that he or she has nothing to give and instead waits to be given to. This may very well be the plight of the child today who is given no encouragement to play, who must mirror the parents rather than the parents mirroring the child, and who is cheered on by the parents to perform tasks that adults want him or her to perform in order to be a successful child.

The correction is simple. Recall the old saying, "All work and no play makes Jack a dull boy." To unspoil childhood we need to bring more play back into children's lives and check our tendencies to reinforce our children only when they are working and never when they are playing. It is not that children's work is not important, but that it cries for a better balance with play if we want our children to be truly successful in life. The task for parents is to facilitate those opportunities and be sensitive to what constitutes "play" for each of their children. One child's painful piano practice is the next child's passionate pleasure. With that in mind, if a child can't find at least an hour a day (and ideally, much more) to get lost in reverie, drama, games, creations, or just plain pleasure or fun, we have an over-worked child.

CHILDREN AND THEIR PARENTS:
THE SHOEMAKER AND THE ELVES

As play leaves the stage of daily life and parents cheerlead only for their children's accomplishments, there is a particular, insidious way that parents take over for the children to ensure their success. With no time to play, and so much work to do, parents worry their children will buckle under the load. Mothers and fathers feel compelled to step in.

A librarian reports a new phenomenon: parents coming to the library to "look things up" for their children, or, more accurately, parents coming to the library to do their children's homework. She reports parents' explanations for appearing at the librarian's desk with grammar school or high school assignments: "My son has football practice"; "Brittany has a gymnastics class"; "It seems like an awful lot of work for a sixth grader." Other parents bring their children with them to the library but then take over, leaving the child to be the silent partner. This is truly a phenomenon of pampering in which the child succeeds without even trying. The librarian blasts these parents as "the ones who are so ambitious for their precious progeny that they end up stunting the kids' learning processes."[8]

Indeed, the outcome for the children may be damaging, thwarting their own development. Parents' library takeovers are a prime example of being too involved and too overzealous for success, not just because of their ambitiousness, but also because of their guilt for the mess they have made for their children. As parents sweep their children up in the same mania that governs their own lives, the children are so overcommitted and overscheduled that they could not possibly attend to all the tasks expected of them in a week. Just as there is no time to parent, there is no time for children to manage all of childhood today. Parents, rather than being able to pull their children out of the rat race, try to compensate by taking over some of the child's load. A silly solution, in the long run, as it undermines the very purpose of homework itself—to train students to work successfully on their own. It also becomes a Herculean task for the parents, who are already typically overworked and overtired, and are now taking on the extra burden of their children's work. But if the trade off is a few hours less sleep for a reduction of a child's stress and an enhancement of a child's success, the parents are all for it.

I think back on my own experience as a parent and compare it to my experience as a child. There is no doubt that I have been more involved in my children's academic work than my parents were in mine. My mother and father gave the three of us, my brothers and me, the clear message that education was important and high effort was both expected and supported. While my older brother and I were still young, my parents purposely relocated to a new community where the public schools were top-notch. The rest was up to us. Their approach appeared to work well. All three of us succeeded in our academic goals and later in our career endeavors.

I, along with my husband, have passed on to our children the same clear message: Education is important, try your best. But all the way through my daughter's college years, I continued to get long-distance calls from her asking for help editing a paper. I now get similar calls from my son. I also admit to having been one of those parents guilty of occasionally running to the library to "help out" one of my overstressed children who had fallen behind in an assignment. Is it just because both my husband and I have higher education degrees and my parents didn't that we find ourselves so much more involved in the children's work than my own parents ever were? I do not think so. I believe it is a generational phenomenon far broader than my own family experience. We ourselves have had the opportunity for achieving so much, and this has spiraled into boundless dreams and expectations for our children. The boundaries between children's "work" and parents' are blurred. Our own worry about our children's future sometimes interferes. Our lack of availability in other ways makes us overeager to involve ourselves where we can—in this case, in the children's academic work.

We are also swayed, either subliminally or directly, by the belief that children's success in the classroom is directly correlated with parents' involvement with their children's academics at home. It is not enough simply to supply the children with an enriching environment; we must be directly involved in their work. In a country in which the public school system is in terrible shape, this may be a very good, if not necessary, strategy on parents' part. But we cannot say parents' involvement is just a function of failing schools, because parents with children in the highest quality private schools are equally, if not more, involved in school assignments as parents of children in the public schools.

The problem is that we step in and do not know when to exit. Certainly some children who are floundering need the monitoring and intervention of their parents to stay on track. But I'm talking about children who could actually being doing much more on their own, if given the chance . . . and the time. With them, it is time to exit when we find we are doing the work *for* our children and they just watch, follow, or wait on the sidelines. It is time to exit when we don't wait for our children to ask for help but just roll up our sleeves and start working. Better to quietly make yourself available and invite your child to solicit your help. And if your children are only too eager to enlist your help, even if they could do it themselves, why not give them a chance to try it first on their own before you step in?

The ultimate goal of parenthood is to enable children to be able to live and function independently, without their parents. Yet in their strong desire to facilitate fame, parents often lose sight of this goal, or of the appropriate means for getting there. Though parents are only too well aware that their children will have to demonstrate competence, confidence, and accomplishment to make it in this world, they can forget the critical component of that equation: competence, confidence, and accomplishment *independently*. It becomes a team effort: "*We* have a paper to finish tonight"; "*We've* been practicing for the recital for months now."

In a society where the immediate family has become the main nucleus of intimacy and "community," this joint effort might be taken as a positive demonstration of a collaborative process in which parents are really there for their children. But more honestly, the behavior is typically fueled by the phenomenon of pampering toward success. Middle-class parents today were typically raised with a confident sense that the best way to guarantee that something is done well is to do it yourself. With that sensibility underlying their strong desire for their children to achieve, it is easy to step in and do it *for* the child, all the while thinking you are doing it *with* the child.

Like the shoemaker, children go to sleep at night and wake up to find their work done for them by the elves, their parents. The difference is that the shoemaker was an overworked and oppressed adult fortunate enough to have elves who altruistically came to his aid, whereas the children, not so obviously downtrodden, might simply be better off left to their own resources so they will learn to sew their own leather. On the other hand, like the shoemaker, perhaps it is true that the children are given more work than they can possibly handle. But rather than becoming elves, parents might better become advocates who aim to reduce the load on their children. Instead parents often accept and even create the over-scheduled lives of their children and then compensate by stepping in to do the work for them.

Intending to ensure children's perfection, parents end up shooting themselves in the foot with their wild vacillations or strange admixtures of pushing and pampering. Their efforts have a boomerang effect as fairy godmothers now become transformed into the shoemakers' elves and end up thwarting the children's independence and opportunities to establish their own competencies.

If there is any critical moment to remind ourselves that we are active agents rather than passive victims of our circumstances, it is around this issue of reducing children's load. We do have other options, such as cutting down the number of extracurricular activities our children are involved in, protesting when schools give more homework than children can handle, stopping ourselves from putting pressure on our children and thinking that well-being equals high performance, period. What we want for our children may not be a good match for who they are. They are little people forming but not yet formed, who need the time and space to "do their own thing" without somebody stepping in to do it for them.

An adolescent with whom I have become acquainted made remarkable progress throughout high school. Despite a fairly significant learning disability, he put his nose to the grindstone and persevered to excel academically. To his parents' credit, they communicated continued support and faith in their son's abilities, despite his learning problems. They also placed a lot of performance demands on him, and grew anxious if he did not respond. Except in one area. Throughout the boy's high school years, his mother typed all of his papers. Now it was time for this boy to leave for college. Computers, word processing, and typing were still foreign to him. What was he to do—bring his mother to college with him? The mother, to ease her son's load and in response to her child's seeming difficulties in mastering use of a keyboard, had stepped in to aid her son. She did the work for him, rather than supporting her son to learn to do it for himself. Granted, with such support this child met with good academic success, but at what price to his independence? Without his mother as personal scribe, he was ill prepared to leave home and stand on his own in a setting that would demand endless typing.

Compare this to a description of adult–child relations in a Native American tribe. In this culture, elder men sit together and discuss local affairs. The children are present, but quiet, perhaps engaged in various domestic tasks. In this context, a grandfather turns and asks his three-year-old granddaughter to close the door. The door is heavy, hard to shut. The little girl attempts to close it, but with no success. The grandfather simply repeats his request to close the door, several times. The other men remain serious and patient until the child finally succeeds in her task. The grandfather then thanks her, communicating that she has done something very special for him. The grown-ups waited patiently, giving the child the time to accomplish her task successfully. They made sure not to push her beyond her means by asking her to do the impossible. They were in no hurry, yet were quite aware of her developing competencies. No one stepped in and took away her own discovery of her ability to succeed in the task and her efficacy in carrying out a responsibility requested of her. There was no great applause at the end, but a simple thank you for doing the job asked of her.[9]

If my adolescent acquaintance could have met up with the measured response of the Native American elders rather than the muddle of pushing and pampering he has received at home, his path to college and independence might be an easier one. It would have been far better for his parents to recognize that he was indeed capable of learning to work a computer and that he would better function, albeit with some sweat and tears, without the constant infusion of his mother's ministrations. Even the most disabled child will benefit from the bolstering of independence and the honing of skills as close as possible to the level of his or her peers, within reasonable and realistic expectations for that child—all done in a low-key way with a minimum of cheers and applause.

If his parents could have made those shifts, he might have avoided the major depression and anxiety about being able to make it on his own anywhere but in the sanctity and safety of his own home and family. His typing experience was emblematic of the many ways his parents both demanded too much but also did too much for him. We see here a prime example of how pampering combined with pushing in the arena of children's achievements can be lethal, fostering false accomplishment and faltering independence.

ALL DRESSED UP WITH NO PLACE TO GO

There is yet another lesson to be learned from the story of the little Native American girl and her elders. The task required of this small girl is very different than the typical achievements set before the typical middle-class child. The little three-year-old was asked to do something very important for her elders. In contrast, middle-class children are often pressured, but not really given anything important to do. Their childhood is basically a long apprenticeship for the future. The children not only make no economic contribution to the society, they do little that is socially relevant. No cows to be driven to the field, no younger ones to be tended to, few household chores to be completed.[10]

D. W. Winnicott talked about the importance of the child developing opportunities for "contributing in." By this he meant the chance to give to others, but more generally, to provide services to those around him or her. He theorized that the desire to do this has its roots in infancy, when the infant experiences anxiety about his or her desires to consume the parent, to take everything from the parent and maybe even destroy what is loved. The small baby is relieved of this anxiety as he or she develops the growing confidence that there will be an opportunity for "reparations," for making it up to the parent and later to the general environment. The reparations take the form of the little child's urge to work or to acquire skills. This is how the child develops confidence that he or she will have opportunities to give something back, to contribute in.[11]

In other words, we all have destructive feelings, as part of the human condition, and those feelings are first directed toward the ones we love most. We move toward health by being given the opportunity to balance those impulses and ideas with constructive "work" and contributions to others. This movement is embedded in children's education in which they develop capacities and skills that are valuable to those around them. It is up to the elders to make sure those opportunities are available. Their efforts will facilitate the beginning of "community involvement."

Children are no doubt busy developing skills or learning to fend for themselves in their parents' absence. But in terms of doing something that contributes in or appears to have some immediate importance to the people around them, the opportunities are slim, if not nonexistent. We might say that children's "work" ranges from being self-directed, solipsistic, and future oriented, to being of no immediate importance whatsoever. We are so focused on preparing for our children's future or placing demands on them to get through the daily hurdles of a hassled, hurried life that we have overlooked one of the most important components of achievement: to know that you are a significant and important contributor to the people around you *now*.

I am reminded of a recent series of events in my community. Across the street from my office in Oakland is a lake and adjoining park. Each June, a festival is held at the lake, targeted at children and families. In June 1994, a riot broke out on the last night of the festival. It involved large groups of teenagers pitted against the police. Afterward, community activists, local officials, and festival planners met to figure out what happened and discuss ways to prevent a reoccurrence in the future. They determined that no events were planned especially for teenagers and young adults, leaving them with nothing to do but get into trouble. In the future, the planners would correct this by providing special programs and activities geared to young people, rather than simply shutting the festival down or moving it to another location, as others in the community had demanded. Even in trying to remedy the problems for youth at the

Festival at the Lake, the organizers could only think about providing fun and pleasure. They failed to consider including the young people by "putting them to work"—contributing to the organizing, set-up, running, or clean-up of the event itself. In this way, children are coddled, neither pushed nor even encouraged to achieve in the "contributing-in" process.

A nine-year-old child may have been pushed to practice for many years so that she is now able to get up and play a beautiful violin piece. Yet that same child may have never done a household task or helped out in any way that was of immediate importance. We push the development of children's skills, but only in a very narrow arena. Academics, sports, and artistic skills flourish in our middle-class children, but at the expense of more "basic" tasks that would allow the child to feel some sense of immediate relevance, such as cooking a simple family meal, helping with the family wash, or teaching younger siblings to tie their shoes.

Even a four-year-old can help put silverware on the table, and a twelve-year-old has the capacity to plan an entire meal, albeit perhaps not one you would choose as the epitome of nutrition and dietary excellence. If we just watch what our children do in their daily lives as they play and interact, we can translate those observed skills and readinesses into tasks that are age appropriate, meaningful, and helpful. If a child is capable of mixing two chemicals to make synthetic rubber in his chemistry set, that same child ought to be able to handle mixing detergent, bleach, and fabric softener in the washing machine.

We may stop and ask, "What about latchkey kids and those left for long hours to fend for themselves while their parents are elsewhere?" True, those children learn some important self-help skills, but with little sense of being part of a community. They certainly help their families out and become citizens-in-the-making by learning how to make a meal for themselves, how to keep the door locked and stay indoors until their parents come home, how to call 911, or in less fortunate families, how to make it out on the streets. But, too often, the responsibilities stop as soon as the parents return home. The children then rarely have the opportunity to experience themselves as part of a collective effort. They know more about fending for themselves when they are on their own, developing individualistic "survival" skills that, in the most immediate sense, benefit no one but themselves.

The default position of parents today regarding their children's rooms is telling in this regard. The new sensibility is, "Well, it's their room, so if they want to keep it like a pigsty that's their prerogative." In the eyes of many a mother and father, it keeps family peace and separates the battles from the wars. The idea that a child's bedroom is also one of the rooms in the family abode and that the child's responsibility is to keep some semblance of order in their small section of the home no longer pertains in many American households. Perhaps we need to rethink this. By asking our children to abide by some modicum of the hygiene and straightening routines applied to the rest of the house, we could send our children a message that they are neither boarders nor royalty exempt from lifting a finger. Rather than their room being their private palace, such a demand could transform our "majesties, the babies" into collective citizens who internalize a self-concept that they are significant contributors to an entity larger than themselves.

Our reluctance to demand our children to pitch in does not stop at messy rooms. At the end of the day, we back off from asking the children to help with dinner and clean up because they have four hours of homework awaiting them or because now it is time for Mom, Dad, and the kids to have some scheduled "quality family time," which precludes work of any kind.

Ironically, we think we are too busy and harried to take the time to train our children to help out. One would think that in a household of harried and overworked people, the parents would feel more driven to get the children to pitch in to lighten the load of household work. But because of parental guilt and because in a time-management crunch it is often easier to get the job done if you do it yourself rather than rely on an untrained apprentice, the child is exempt. Unfortunately, this stance simply feeds into the myth that our children have nothing important to provide and could do nothing to ease everyone's load.

Children quickly internalize this sensibility about themselves. I recall a teenager who had herself adopted the no-work stance. She told me her mother was out of her mind to think she would have time to clear the table and wash the dishes, given volley ball, homework, and piano practice. How could her mother not realize that she was entitled to an exemption from such responsibilities? She wasted not a minute letting her mother know that, and sure enough, her mother backed off in her demands.

If children are too busy or harried to have the time to chip in, perhaps we need to rethink the balance of their life to create more time for just such contributing-in activities. The entitled attitude of princes and princesses is no more attractive than overworked, over-stressed sons and daughters. A little less afterschool activity and a little more family or community service might make a more empathic and well-rounded person.

But what about the swelling ranks of young people who take on paid work? The number of adolescents holding part-time jobs has skyrocketed in the past decade. Teens today are twice as likely to work as in 1950. More than five million young people ages twelve to seventeen now work, according to a recent survey.[12] It would make sense that, in an era of major recessions and high inflation, individuals would begin getting jobs at an earlier age. The perk is that teenagers finally get the opportunity to work at something that makes them part of the larger social order. But the vast majority of teenagers are not saving their earnings for their future or contributing to the household income. The teenager typically gets a job to have more spending money—the earnings are used for the child's own leisure time activities, clothes, entertainment, transportation. *Newsweek* reports: "While Wally Cleaver's afternoons were occupied by varsity track, basketball and hanging around with Eddie Haskell, Brandon Walsh on 'Beverly Hills, 90210' waits on tables at the Peach Pit because his wealthy parents think it will teach him responsibility—and so that he could buy a Mustang convertible."[13] Brandon may indeed be learning responsibility, but he contributes only to himself, rather than to the family, some "larger cause," or some future goal, such as a college fund. And if he is like other teenagers who hold jobs while attending school, he can also expect his grades to fall and his responsibility for schoolwork to flounder, undermining the very achievement his parents have been priming him for.

The only way middle-class children today are engaged in the "contributing-in" process so important to development is by providing themselves as the object of their parents' love and demonstrating to all around them that they are successful in their progression through the stages of childhood and toward adulthood. Superstars in certain areas, we actually leave our children retarded in others. In the meantime, they become commodities whose main contribution is to be happy and accomplished. As they grow to expect that this should be their position in life, we may actually be contributing to their inability to function when they discover that they are not as accomplished as they would like to be, as happy as their parents would like them to be, or as important to the world as they have been primed to believe they are.

Few parents are unfamiliar with the child's accusatory, "Why should I bother learning _____ , it's such a waste." We know the proper response, "Someday you'll find it very useful and that's why it's important to work at it now."; or "It's part of becoming a well-rounded, educated person." But perhaps our children would protest less if we balanced our focus on their preparation for the future with achievements that count *now,* even if they are as minor as closing a heavy door for the elders. If we can do that, we can avoid dressing our children for success and then giving them no place to go.

REMEDYING THE FALLOUTS
FROM PUSHING AND PAMPERING

We have enough evidence of what happens to children who are pumped for success and loved primarily for those successes. The children feel perpetually pressured to be adaptable, adept, and outstanding in their abilities. But they end up lacking any core of their own. They can lose their vitality and spontaneity. They may even be at risk for either narcissistic or depressive disorders. They come to overrely on the admiration of others as they mature, or they may discover the emptiness of their accomplishments and the impossibility of ever receiving love just for who they are, rather than what they do.[14] In a sense, they develop a "false self."

This is certainly not what we have in mind for our children in wanting to build their self-esteem and ensure their success. And most of us are not so extreme that we would demand that our children become our mirror, performing only for us, with their job in life being to reflect back our own bolstered self-esteem through their successes. But as we get caught up in pushing and then pampering our children toward success, the story of the "false self" child provides a cautionary tale.

There are many steps we can take so our children do not develop "false selves." By this I mean inauthentic ways of being and acting designed, consciously or unconsciously, to please those around them. This would be in direct contrast to expressions of their true thoughts, feelings, and desires, which would be the key components of a "true self." The false self is ten-year-old Jonathan saying, "Thank you very much, Dr. Ehrensaft . . . and I'm so looking forward to going to the opera with my mother." The true self is Jonathan months into therapy racing around the room on hands and knees laughing and squealing as he tries to grab my leg in stuffed-animal baseball.

Children do best when they are allowed to unfold at their own speed rather than being forced to adapt to their parents' expectations for achievement. Following this principle will help a child's true self flourish and greatly reduce the risks of a "false self" outcome. Holding back the excessive applause is equally important, as the perpetual cheerleading only highlights for the child the need to adapt to the parents' hopes and expectations for outstanding behavior, as children typically do want to please their parents and see that reflected in their parents' joy. If we can come to see more clearly our children's genuine needs for a less pressured trajectory through childhood, the children will be released from the syndrome of worry that their parents will not respect them if they do not make it to the top and the constant pressure that they must always be the best, never having a failure, never being out of sorts.

The baby in the cartoon asked for a sabbatical from flash cards. Real live children can tell you in all kinds of ways that the priming for success is not working. They are capable of sit-down strikes in the face of their parents' undue achievement expectations or excessive applause. They can communicate in more subtle ways, getting distracted, listless, hyperactive, irritable, or anxiety ridden. As they grow older they can reach the conclusion, "I'll have none of this for me," when confronted with their parents' own driven and harried high-achieving lives. We need to listen very carefully to these messages that even our very young children may be sending out. Such behaviors tell us that being a superstar pumped up for fame but with nowhere important to go is bringing our children stress but no happiness and needs to be remedied.

In 1994, I ran a workshop for parents in which I asked them to write an incident in which they felt at their wits' end with their child. Here is a response from one of the workshop participants:

> My son is a high school senior, 17½ years old. He's been very hard working, a successful student and athlete. In choosing a college for next year, he's always felt very strongly about specifically which ones he wanted—especially because he only wanted to compete athletically in certain programs. We disagreed, but went along. He was heavily recruited by some of the top schools in the country, an enviable position. But in the last few weeks, he's talked about not really wanting to compete at college at all. This has always been his choice and his dream. Now we have to decide whether to encourage him to not compete or help him get over his "burn-out" and go on to compete.

"His choice," "his dream," "burn-out." Could it be that all of his hard work was not for himself but to earn the favor of his parents? Could it be that his parents did too much of the work for him, leaving him ill prepared for the world of independence awaiting him? If he is burning out, what is the source of the stress? Is this the crash that comes from a realization of the inauthenticity of his striving? Is he afraid that he can't really do it or is he ambivalent about wanting to? And is his parents' confusion about whether to *encourage* his retreat or *push* his pursuit emblematic of a conflict in parenting that has gone on for years in this family? None of these questions could be adequately answered without carefully interviewing each of the parties involved. But the scenario of the youthful overachiever who suddenly retreats when faced with the "big time" is an allegory of our times.

If his parents, or any of us, for that matter, had the opportunity to play with these questions, given all that we now know about pushing and pampering, they might have avoided the predicament they now find themselves in. The "competing in college," which I suspect was metaphorical for competing *at all*, might not have become such a charged issue for this boy. Now faced with the dilemma, it is still not too late to remedy the situation. I would encourage the parents to back off and let this young man make his own decision about competing in college.

We need to push our children less, allow them to play more, applaud them less, and allow them to do more on their own while at the same contributing in more to others. Why? Because if we can do so, we will remedy the two main psychological fall outs for the child who has been both pushed and pampered: a decrease in authenticity and an increase in generalized anxiety.

As long as we foster such inauthenticity and anxiety by our swings between pushing and pampering, the child is robbed of a true self and, more specifically, of developing the capacity for play and ultimately for creativity. Not only parents' *conscious* devaluation of play but specific *unconscious* transmissions from parent to child in the muddle of pushing and pampering debilitate the development of a child's capacity to play. The beginning of play in the first year of life is predicated on the capacity to be alone in the presence of another, to be able to sit at the feet of a trusted adult, engaged in one's own reveries, but subtly aware of the safe "environment" created by that adult. From birth on children are given little opportunity for that type of space today. Put very bluntly, there is always someone in their face. Both pushed and pampered, children never get the opportunity just to be alone *and* unencumbered—within a "holding environment"—so as to experience the power of their own "stuff." When they are alone, it is often in the absence of a safe environment. When they *are* in the presence of another, they are seldom given the opportunity to be alone. We need to turn that around. Not just parents, but society as a whole must work to make the world safer and the child more connected to that world. As parents, we can try to be there more than we are, if we have that option, and when there, give our children space to be alone and experience themselves—in our presence.

The plight of the toddler/doctor is movingly told in a clinical tale. Some years ago, an adolescent whom I was seeing in therapy as a result of his anxieties about his school performance came to one of his sessions wracked with worry and furious with himself, because, he said, "I left my retainer in the Waldorf-Astoria." In the course of his treatment, Malcolm's parents had unexpectedly separated, sending Malcolm into an emotional tailspin. He had channeled his worries into his pervasive performance anxieties. He could not chastise himself enough for having been so irresponsible as to lose his orthodontic retainer in his room at the posh hotel in New York where he and his mother had just vacationed. Further, his orthodontist was going to be terribly angry with him that he had not kept up with his orthodontia, because, after all, it is impossible to wear a retainer that is lost in the Waldorf-Astoria. Malcolm imagined that he was going to have to start all over wearing braces. Having messed up on his retainer, his head started spinning with all the other things he might start messing up. He hadn't yet finished his school reports, which were due several weeks hence. There was no way he was ever going to get into college unless he stayed up all night writing them. If he didn't get into a decent college, he would never receive entrance into medical school. And if he didn't get into medical school, he might as well kiss his life good-bye. All because he had left his retainer in the Waldorf-Astoria.

Malcolm's story illustrates the plight of the middle-class child who has been both pushed and pampered. We may feel little sympathy for Malcolm's distress if we compare it to the waking nightmare of the young Rwandan refugee fleeing his homeland amidst the dead and the dying. But Malcolm's spiraling of anxiety, self-castigation, and performance pressure captures the burdens placed on the over-indulged but highly pressured children of today. They have no opportunity just to do nothing. Their parents not only guide but sometimes actually control or shape their every move toward success. Rather than a silver spoon in their mouths, they constantly worry about a retainer that could get lost.

If we go back to the notion of "my toddler, the doctor," and do a play on words by turning them around to make "my doctor, the toddler," we grasp the real contradiction of the concept in the context of pushing and pampering: a catapulting through childhood but a childhood arrest at the same time. By pushing children to accelerate their development, we force them to leave childhood behind prematurely. We can imagine creating a future adult who is in constant search of the "lost child" within, or who feels like he or she has to go back and recapture something that never happened. At the same time, by taking shortcuts to success through serving as elves to our little shoemakers and fairy godparents to their budding self-esteem, we deprive children of the true stepping stones to adulthood and leave them in a constant search for the adults that they are supposed to become. So, indeed, the contradictory toddler/doctor evolves into a lifelong syndrome, rather than just a childhood problem.

Throughout this chapter, I have urged parents and the society at large to find something important for our children to do that is appropriate to their age and makes a difference *now*. I have asked us to stop all the stars and clapping, instead giving quiet but proud recognition for the accomplishments our children genuinely achieve. I have argued for increased time and space for play, and less singular emphasis on our children's cognitive precocity. I have encouraged us to stop being the elves to our shoemakers, and instead do things *with*, but not *for* our child. I have suggested that it would be better, at times, to stop paving the way to our children's success and instead let our children cut their own path and face their own disappointments, being there to help them when they trip but not preventing every fall. Through these measures we can eliminate the risk of the lifelong syndrome of "my toddler, the doctor; my doctor, the toddler." In its place, we can facilitate for our children a healthy integration of productivity and creativity.

CHAPTER SEVEN

· · · · · ·

Parents Bartering
for Love

*Yes, young people may not like us when we set
rules and standards, and that is too bad. When we
worry about our children liking us, however, we
put our needs ahead of our children's needs. When
we try to be pals to our children instead of parents,
we deprive them of their most important source of
internal rules, limits, standards, and controls.*
—DAVID ELKIND[1]

Madeline was seven years old. Distraught that her mother was angry
with her, she yelled out, "You hate me, you hate me!" Christina,
Madeline's mother, tried to reassure her, "No, I love you. I just don't
like what you did." That went nowhere. Madeline screamed back,
"No, you hate me." Christina tried a different tack: "Madeline, don't
you sometimes get angry at me for something I did?" Madeline
paused for a second, then said, "Yeah, of course." Christina rejoined,
"Well, don't you still love me then?" Madeline, with not a moment's
hesitation: "No, I hate you then."

We have just walked in on an interchange in "bartering for love."
The perspective Christina attempted to impart to her daughter was
a sound one: a lesson in separating hated acts from the bonds of love.
From the developmental stance of a seven-year-old, Madeline's perspective was equally sound: If I don't like what you do, then I don't
like you. Madeline was not conceptually ready to differentiate
responses to discrete acts from deeper emotional bonds.

All this would be fine if Christina and all of her cohort group of parents today did not crumble in the face of such retorts from their children. We have a problem: Madeline's perspective is increasingly internalized by grown-ups. If we are displeased with our children, maybe that means we really do not love them. More importantly, if we do something to displease our children, we run the risk that they will stop loving us. Then we might lose them.

A major problem in parenting today is the new trade off between love and respect. For our parents and grandparents, respect, not love, was what was expected from their children. A good child was a well-behaved child, and a good parent was one whose children showed the proper deference to their mother and father, looked up to them, and accepted their parents' guidance without protest. Today, as the boundaries between adulthood and childhood have blurred and as democracy has replaced autocracy in child-rearing norms, it is no longer respect, but *love* that parents seek from their children. Their child's love for them is no longer considered unconditional, as in previous generations, but is now perceived as conditional love, love that can be granted or retracted. This marks an enormous cultural and psychological shift in parenting, unprecedented in earlier generations.

A good parent now becomes the parent who has a child who loves him or her. A bad parent is one who has lost that love or has never secured it. A good parent acquires that love by respecting their child. We no longer demand respect (indeed, we sometimes let our children punch and kick us and call us terrible names). Instead we feel compelled to *give* it. To achieve this, we are led by the misguided notion that we must concentrate on gratifying and never depriving our children. Otherwise, our children will fail to love us. So the old formula, children give respect, parents give the love has gone through a total reversal. Now parents give the respect, children give the love.

In that context, the grown-up dilemma of risking loss of our children's love by expressing displeasure to our children, depriving them, or suggesting that we disrespect them becomes extremely painful and constitutes what I am referring to as the new "bartering for love." We need to release ourselves from this new mind set of respect traded for love, which is fueled so strongly by our parenting by guilt and which leads us unwittingly into relationships where our children, rather than us, seem to be running the show.

WHO IS LOSING WHOM?

In both developmental and psychoanalytic theory, paradigms are developed to explain how a child attaches to another human being early in life. A particular body of work, based on psychoanalytic object relations theory, conceptualizes the internal experiences of a young infant in becoming a "relational" person capable of love and emotional commitment. In the object relations formulation, two major milestones occur in this process of relational development: (1) fear of the loss of the love *object* and (2) fear of the loss of the *love* of the love object.

At the beginning of life, the newborn has no idea that when Mother and Father leave the room they still exist. Regarding both people and inanimate objects, the guiding principle for the tiny infant is "out of sight, out of mind." The baby also lives with the delusional fantasy that she or he has omnipotent control to *make* people appear just by wishing them there.

Then at about six months of age, the infant develops the understanding that people come and go, but when they go they still exist. Maturation and learning force the infant to relinquish the fantasy of magical powers that wish parents into existence. If moms and dads or stable caretakers can pick themselves up and go away, then baby stands the risk of losing them, maybe just when baby wants them. This makes baby nervous, as manifested in either separation anxiety or stranger anxiety. Infants do not want to lose the persons who have now become very important to their survival, and they do not want those persons replaced by anyone else. This angst has been labeled "fear of the loss of the object."[2]

As time goes on, the baby develops increasing autonomy, independence, and motor abilities. Sometimes baby wants to go out and explore or forage on his or her own. Sometimes baby can even feel exasperated with Mom, Dad, or a loved one, and not really want to be around them. By the beginning of the second year of life, baby begins to realize that if he or she has those feelings, maybe Mom or Dad does, too. The baby is now faced with a dilemma: If I want to be my own little person and leave you, maybe you will want to leave me, too.[3] Baby notices that even when a loved one is physically there, the loved one may not be *emotionally* all there. Or, alternatively, the loved one may exude negative feelings while physically there. Just at the time when baby is excited about trying out his or her new wings, a new feeling will soon follow: In my flight I might lose the love of the people I love. This is what is referred to as "the fear of the loss of the love of the object." It is part and parcel of the journey toward caring about others.

As development ensues, the child works through these fears and comes to a feeling by adulthood, if all goes well, that love is a fairly stable state of feeling and being that occurs even when the loved one is not physically present or when the loved one is angry or when one chooses to be alone rather than with the loved one. This is the sensibility that Christina was trying to impart to her daughter. Life events such as divorce, death, or a "falling out" with a close friend or relative can disrupt this stable sense of love and catapult us back into raw feelings of fear of loss of the love of the object and the even more simple fear of loss of the object itself. But with time and opportunity to recuperate and reconsolidate ourselves, we can anticipate getting back on track developmentally in our understandings and experiences of love.

The problem with parenting today is that there has been a reversal in the players in these two concepts. We still see family members worrying that a loved one might stop loving them or perhaps never did. We also see family members worrying that a loved one might actually be lost to them. But the casting of characters in the developmental drama has changed. Now the *parents,* not the infants, become the main players, the protagonists who worry that their children may no longer love them or that they may lose their children altogether. Although the bases of the parents' fears are clearly very different than those of the young child's, the fact remains that the tables have turned, so that we now see parents far outweighing the children in their fears of loss.

What accounts for the parents' worries? First, just as the infant is not sure that Mom or Dad is really there forever, parents today do not trust that their child will be theirs forever. In the contemporary world of family dissolution and single parenthood, one's child is often the only permanent connection an adult can count on. But even that tie is tenuous. Increasingly, children have the chance to "choose" which parent to reside with after a divorce. In extreme situations, a postdivorce child will even refuse to see a parent, either because of tension with that parent or loyalty to the other parent. In many instances, it is not the child but the court that plays its hand in limiting access of a parent to a child following a divorce. Not just divorced parents, but all parents are affected by this new phenomenon of children choosing their parents or parents losing their children.

In 1992, a legal case broke in Florida in which a twelve-year-old boy, Gregory Kingsley, went to court with independent counsel to request termination of parental rights of his biological mother so that he could be adopted by his foster parents. He requested termination on the grounds that his mother had abused and neglected him for most of his life. The final ruling was in his favor. The case, aired on national TV, mesmerized the entire nation. Some of my own little patients came in asking if they too could "divorce" their parents. Their queries were clearly shaped by the media's slant on this case. In a matter of days headlines such as the following appeared in newspapers across the country: "Boy's Bid to 'Divorce' Mom," "12-Year-Old Wins 'Divorce' from Parents," and to alleviate the public anxiety, " 'Divorce' from Mother Not a Likely Trend-Setter."[4]

In the trial, Gregory testified that he "did not love her [his biological mother] as a mother." His success in terminating the parental rights of his mother became broadly disseminated public information. The suit led to criticism by many that such allowable legal actions by children would unleash a rash of frivolous claims by unhappy children to "divorce" their parents. Although legal experts assured the American public that the Kingsley suit was a very extreme case that would never open the floodgates of whimsical termination suits by disgruntled progeny, the experts may have overlooked the real impact of Gregory Kingsley's legal victory on parents today.

I was floored by the number of anxious parents coming into my office shaken by the implications of Gregory's "divorce," particularly parents who had endured or were anticipating child custody disputes with estranged spouses. I watched parents pause and give thought to the actual permanence of their children. The rarity of the case and the legal particularities got lost in the highlighting of the "divorce" phenomenon. Parents were alerted to a change in the currents of history toward enhanced children's rights and increased intervention of government and legal authorities in family life. This cultural shift coalesced with parents' own psychological misgivings that their children may want to leave them and may not love them.

In our society, we underscore the commodity of love. We don't take love as a given, it is something we have to strive for. Once we acquire it, we can also lose it. We want as much of it as we can get. It is even conceivable that we can buy it. Such love, conditional rather than unconditional, can pervade our relationships with our spouses, with our friends, with our own parents. It also extends to relationships with our children. In this trade in love, the threat to the permanency of the parent–child bond through "divorce" is not an easy pill for parents to swallow.

But "divorce" is not the only thing making parents worry about the security of their child's bond to them. Modern psychology has alerted us to the notion that children not only love their parents, they also reject them. In past eras when it was perceived that children's actual physical existence depended on their parents' goodwill, it did not occur to people that children would ever reject their parents, for without the parents' ministrations the children would surely die. But now that children are not so dependent on their parents for survival, the bond is more primarily an emotional one. No longer holding on for their lives, it becomes conceivable that our children could turn from us, not want or even need us anymore. With our new psychological insights about children's rejection, we are ripe for seeing any negative behavior on the child's part as a signal that we are being rejected.[5] So when three-year-old Lily marches off to her room because Mommy hasn't tied her hairbow properly and screams that she has the meanest mommy in the world and wishes she could have a new one, Mommy now agonizes that maybe she has indeed failed as a mother and maybe Lily will reject her in favor of some other adult who is better at fixing hairbows.

On occasion a child's negative behaviors may actually indicate a rejection of the parent, but such a scenario is infinitely more rare than worried parents today have come to believe. More likely, the child is simply registering "I don't like what's happening right now." So why are we ripe for such worry?

With the shift of feeling from unconditional to conditional love in child–parent relationships, it makes sense that parents would be hypervigilant to the signs of rejection from their offspring. But their worry is further fueled by their own internal guilt that they have neither the time to spend nor the resources to call upon to provide their children with a safe, secure, and loving life. It is the same worry that propels them to want the perfect child, the same worry that shapes "my toddler, the doctor."

When individuals serving others feel they are not doing a good enough job, they become ripe for sensitivity to rejection, particularly by the people they are supposed to serve. In the case of parents today, those people are our children. We worry very much that they will not love us because we cannot give them enough reasons to love us. We're not there when we should be or when they want us to be. We're spread too thin. We feel we cannot promise them a good life. All of this leaves us perpetually shaky in our self-assessment as a "good enough parent."

We used to talk about "throw-away" children, children no longer wanted or loved by their parents. Now we fear the potential for "throw-away" parents, mothers and fathers discarded by their children because *they*, the parents, are no longer loved or wanted. In parents' anxious fantasies, the new "kinderdults," when catapulted to their adult-like mode, hold the capacity and are granted the power to inflict such seeming damage on their parents.

Granted, the psychological effect of children creating throw-away parents pales in comparison to the effects on the millions of abused and neglected children so discarded by their mothers and fathers. Yet the threat feels substantial, and it contorts parents' attitudes and behaviors toward fearing the loss of the object, that is, their child. To avoid such an outcome, parents abide by the first tenet in bartering for love: Whatever it takes to assure that I do not lose you, I will do.

In day-to-day life, more pernicious than fear of losing the child completely is parents' gnawing anxiety that they will lose not their child, but their child's love. Recently, Jane, a fifteen-year-old girl, ran away from home. This was quite a jolt to her parents, Paul and Victoria, who were both high-powered professionals with a strong public presence in the community. Secure and firm in their interactions with colleagues, they were just the opposite at home. Always they worried about being good enough parents, always they felt too scattered to ever be good enough parents. Prior to her departure, Paul and Victoria had allowed Jane to stay out until all hours of the night or not come home at all. They did not want to put any reins on her behavior because they feared she would stop loving them if they did. The irony is that they not only lost her love but also her.

They confirmed their worst fears by holding back from doing the very thing that would assure their child that they loved her, ensure that their child would still be there to love, and facilitate the love they were so afraid of losing. If they could have stopped to ask themselves what this child really needed and whether their fears of losing her love were in any way grounded in reality, this story might have taken quite a different turn. It appeared that Jane was communicating in a thousand different ways that she wanted her parents to take notice of her and stop her from doing what she was incapable of stopping on her own. When she called to announce that she was not coming home for the night, her hope was that her parents would take the reins and say, "Absolutely not, you be home by 11 P.M." *That* would have shown that they loved her and would not let her put herself in risky situations. *That* message would have let her know that her parents were really there for her, rather than transmitting to her their own anxieties about whether she was going to be there for them. If they had known that they had the option to set firmer limits and keep closer tabs on Jane, they might have avoided having a runaway daughter. This more "interventionist" tactic, rather than their helpless, laissez-faire attitude, would have better served as the epoxy of love and stopped Jane, not from not loving, but from feeling desperately unloved.

To help families like Jane's, "Tough Love" programs have sprung up all around the country, programs targeting parents of out-of-control adolescents to teach them limit- and boundary-setting skills and help them over either their inhibitions or negligence in providing appropriate guidelines for their children. Just the title, "Tough Love," underscores the trouble parents today may be having with parent–child love, trouble with a prescribed remedy of transforming "soft/weak" into "tough" love.

In the meantime, we continue to be driven by the fear that the parent who is not good enough will not be loved enough. Governed by such fear, we succumb to the second tenet in bartering in love: I'll do whatever I need to do to assure that you will keep loving me, because there are a lot of good reasons why you might not love me.

We can clearly see this second tenet in action when we watch how parents today handle separations from their children. It is natural for small children to cling and protest when a parent is about to leave. A parent may then draw the conclusion that their child's clinging and protest is a clear indicator that they have done something wrong. With that conclusion, they construe that the best remedy is to stay home or take the child with them wherever they are going. Again and again, parents come to me for consultation with this very problem: Their child is "tortured" by their leave-takings. Should they stop going out anymore, except when they have to?

In their attempt to grant the child whatever the child is demanding to assure that the child will not withdraw love, I watch these parents get blinded to the natural and inevitable process of sons and daughters working out their anxieties about relationships through expressing their childhood fears about losing their parent or their parent's love. Granted, situations occur where children are overtaxed, asked to endure too frequent separations for too long a time at too early an age. In such cases, their strong and persistent protests must be listened to very carefully, with adjustments made to alleviate their anxieties. But I am not referring to those cases. Instead, I am talking about the transitory protests by a child who is not so overly taxed. These protests, although potentially very intense, typically die down within minutes after the final good-bye. The child is then happily engaged in whatever comes next, except, of course, if he or she has picked up on the parents' own anxieties about the leave-taking, as when a parent comes back five times to say a final good-bye or leaves with a worried, anxious expression and a false assurance that they will only be gone a minute.

I watch parents respond to these transitory protests to separations by focusing on how they themselves have not been loving or attentive enough. They imagine that the separation from their child was a terrible mistake. They vow never to repeat it again. In their own minds not only may they have permanently damaged their child's fragile psyche; their child may also hate them for their actions.

In these situations, the reparative work involves addressing parents' second tenet in the bartering for love—I'll do whatever it takes to keep you loving me. First I assess whether the child is exhibiting excessive clinginess or anxiety that signals that the child is in trouble and needs some extra attention. If the child is, we attend to that, perhaps reducing the number or length of separations or finding better ways to facilitate them when they need to happen. The latter might involve building in some quiet, relaxed time before the separation, leaving the child with a note or picture as a "transitional object," limiting the length of the separation, and making sure a trusted adult is present who can comfort the child.

If it appears that the protests are transitory, normal, and not to be backed away from, I invite the parents to think about what the child's clinging or crying means and how they might respond. When the child clings to Mother or Father's ankle and pleads, "Don't go," he or she may well be communicating not that the parents have failed or done something wrong, but that he or she loves them enough to take notice of their leaving. If they always give in to their child's protests, are they doing it to help their child or to assuage their own agonizing guilt? Do they unwittingly send their child a message that he or she is too weak or fragile to cope with time away from a parent? The path to love is not through removing every thorn in a child's way. Frustration and pain are part and parcel of healthy growing, if experienced in correct doses and with parental support to get the child through. If we block all our children's frustrations, we inhibit their growth. Each time a child successfully masters a separation and discovers the stability of the relationship—Mom and Dad do come back—the child moves one step forward in the developmental progression toward a feeling of stable love that transcends time and place. Shifting our mindset to the idea that, nine times out of ten, the separation protests are only momentary and life quickly resumes a happy note with the baby-sitter or day care provider is a surer remedy than canceling all further outings until further notice.

What is the consequence when baby *and* parent are *both* worried about losing each other or each other's love? By middle childhood, it looks like the tables are turned, with parent as the grant*ee* agonizing about the shakiness of the bond and child the grant*or* holding the power to give or retract love. This is a losing proposition for all parties involved. Child suffers from the lack of a strong holding environment with appropriate boundary setting in which mother and father are confident in their ties to the child and the child can grow secure that parents will always be there, both physically and emotionally. In their panic about love, parents forfeit the opportunity to receive their child's respect, and instead are frantically trying to give it. In the process, they end up denying their children a strong and good figure to look up to.

With all their worrying, parents are robbed of the comfort of "undying love" that gives us permission to relax a little and feel confident that, even in the face of minor or occasionally major mistakes, we will still have the love of our child, despite our imperfection as parents. If we can claim that gift, we can alleviate the pounding anxiety that ensues when we are constantly walking on eggshells in our ministrations to our children.

TO GRATIFY OR DEPRIVE? THAT IS THE QUESTION

"A Tale of Two Mothers," an article published in the magazine *Working Mother*,[6] is the story of the tensions between a working mother and a stay-at-home mother. These two women were friends. One stayed home with the children, while the other had a paid job. Each worried about the outcomes for their own children. The working mother worried that her children were too independent. The stay-at-home mother worried that her children were not independent enough. The working mother thought that perhaps her children were too materialistic because they had been showered with material goods, both out of parental guilt and because their family could afford it with their two incomes. The stay-at-home mother observed her already grown children and worried they too were overly materialistic in reaction to growing up with economic deprivation in a one- rather than two-paycheck family.

Each mother struggled with a basic concern plaguing most parents today: What is gratifying and what is depriving? Do we gratify our children when we buy them a lot of things or do we deprive them of the opportunity to appreciate the finer, more esoteric things in life? Do we gratify our children's need for nurturance and companionship by being home with them everyday, or do we deprive them of the opportunity to establish autonomy and self-help skills? Never has a generation been so confused about the difference between gratification and deprivation and never has a generation been so obsessed with worry that they fall too far at one end of the spectrum or the other. And, in truth, never has a generation vacillated so greatly between gratification and deprivation in their child-rearing behavior.

In the Victorian era, the mode of child rearing in vogue emphasized deprivation rather than gratification—early toilet training, no masturbation, no sex, no aggression. Freud came along and his theories had a tremendous impact in changing that emphasis. He demonstrated how damaging such deprivation could be to a child's psyche. The Freudian tradition led to sanctions for more progressive and permissive child rearing, with far greater emphasis on gratification than on deprivation. Many believe that the height of this new permissiveness in child rearing occurred in the post-World War II period, first marked by the publication of Dr. Spock's *Baby and Child Care* in 1946, a book that has since sold more copies than the Bible. The shift toward permissiveness and gratification was accompanied by a cultural belief that no one should ever have to suffer—either adult or child.

The swing from deprivation to gratification as a cornerstone in child rearing has been neither simple nor linear. For some, the emphasis on gratification was taken to excess and was read to mean that the child should be allowed to do anything. The "free school" movement instigated by the work of Neill at Summerhill in the 1960s exemplifies gratification at its extreme. I am reminded of a visit I made in the early 1970s to a free school in Montreal. I came just to observe. A boy, about ten years old, wanted to make a phone call to his parents to say where he would be after school. Some other boys were playing with the phone. The boy explained that he needed to use the phone to call his parents. The other boys paid no heed. Each time he would go for the phone, they would play with the rotary dial or grab the receiver. They were having a good time. The boy finally gave up and walked away, defeated and deflated. No adult intervened. The other boys' gratification became this boy's victimization under the principle of "doing your own thing."

Free schools and the accompanying "do your own thing" ideology have become anachronisms of the 1960s. Since then people have landed on some middle ground that recognizes the need for a better balance between gratification and deprivation. It is now clear that a life without at least a modicum of imposed "deprivations" becomes anarchic chaos, a solipsistic drama the likes of *The Lord of the Flies*. Applied to child rearing, children should not be free to do whatever they want whenever they want. It is not even clear that they want to. Instead, it appears that they depend on their parents to build structures around them that are appropriately measured, both to free children's desires but also to bind them so that the children do not get carried away. In my clinical practice, I explain it to parents with the metaphor that children need to know that somebody with a driver's license is driving the bus so the bus doesn't careen out of control.

As a reaction to the dominant trend toward gratifying the children, we see a glimmer of change as when Ronald Taffel, child-rearing columnist for *McCall's* magazine, writes: "People don't want to go back to the old ways of the pre-psychology era with its repression and oppression, but the excesses of the child-centeredness that created a generation of kids out of control doesn't work either. What you're seeing is a swing back to some kind of middle ground where there is a greater respect for creating a sense of structure that at the same time doesn't squash the spirit of children."[7] But we're all desperately struggling to find that balance point, lured always toward the side of overgratifying.

The pull toward gratification is particularly strong in the context of bartering for love because of our cultural belief that love is built on the foundation of satisfied desires. In parent–child bonds this translates to keeping our children happy and making sure their every need and want is fulfilled. But that does not mean we will really be doing right by our children. A child with completely satisfied needs, with nothing to want for, is left bereft of desire and devoid of frustration tolerance, and parents who work to ensure the bonds of love by satisfying every one of their child's needs and avoiding any kind of unhappiness are like machines working overtime, racing toward collapse.

Pamela and Gordon believed that a crying child meant a failing parent. As a small baby, their son, Richard, was given a warm and enriched environment. He had two parents who anticipated his every need and quietly removed obstacles from his course before he ever knew they were in his way. In his early months, this was appropriate behavior on his parents' part, and it seemed to pay off. He had a bucolic and blissful first couple of years, and a fairly peaceful third year as well. His parents remained attuned to his every need. Richard smiled most of the time and Pamela and Gordon felt full and happy as parents. They all seemed to have found nirvana.

But then it was time for Richard to attend preschool. Nirvana quickly turned to purgatory. Pamela and Gordon, in their strong commitment to being the best parents they could be and with their staunch belief that the best way to do this was through gratifying Richard, missed the boat. They failed to present their son with the "gradual failures" that would allow him to function in the world. They failed to understand that limit setting and letting Richard find his own way out of a situation were supposed to be the next items on the agenda in helping Richard move forward as a confident, lovable, and loved preschooler. They just kept providing and providing. As a result, Richard was not accustomed to "failures in attunement." He did not comprehend why his every need was not met at school by his teacher of ten children, as it was at home. His conflict-free home life existed in stark contrast to his new battlefield at school. Soon the battles were carried home. No one was happy anymore. In the concerted effort to keep Richard satisfied and gratified, Richard was deprived of the basic tools that would help him cope in the world—patience, waiting his turn, dealing with frustration, problem solving, hoping for something better.

Pamela and Gordon came to me deflated and disorganized. They couldn't understand why their regime of "sensitive parenting" had misfired. I asked them how each of them would feel if the other one catered to every one of their needs and anticipated their every want. Would they really like that? Pamela said she would feel suffocated, Gordon groaned that it would be like living with his mother again. I asked them to consider whether Richard was really all that different. Even though he seemed to clamor for such attention, at the same time he was no longer happy when he got it. Perhaps he had outgrown that early blissful period when everyone circles around us, and was now longing for something different.

I asked them to do an experiment. They were to pick something that he was balking about doing on his own at preschool and that they always did for him at home. They both immediately agreed it was putting on his socks and slip-on shoes, which was causing big battles at school after naptime. With good spirit they were to ask him to start doing it on his own. When he came crying for help, their task was first to encourage him to keep trying on his own. If he grew frustrated or furious, they could tell him, "We know it's very hard but we really think you can handle it." They were to hold back from jumping in to gratify his demands to do it for him. They were to try if for a week and report back.

It wasn't so easy—Richard ranted like a caged bear for the first few days, furious at the loss of home services. But to Pamela and Gordon's credit, they stuck with it, and had a child who was a happy self-dresser within a couple of weeks. This was their first step on a longer path of putting greater demands on Richard, fueled with the new insight that it was not harming but helping him when they thwarted some of his wants and allowed him to work through his own disappointments and frustrations. As Richard was able to discover that deprivation once in a while wasn't really such a bad thing, he settled down into his preschool life, and rather than either nirvana or purgatory, a more down-to-earth, peaceful era ensued both at home and at school. The love ties between Pamela, Gordon, and Richard were in no way damaged; in fact, they actually seemed stronger.

Sometimes parents come to me and complain, "Nothing I'm doing seems to be working. I give her everything she wants, and then she still isn't happy, and just asks for something else." Often this will happen when parents are desperately trying to compensate for an assault on the child's well-being, as when there's been a marital separation. The parents grow angry at their child for being an ingrate, after all they have done. They are correct in registering that their child is unhappy, but they may be missing the message. Their child is trying to tell them to give it up—their eager attempts to secure love by gratifying and gratifying aren't working.

To continue the example of divorce, children are typically miserable when their parents separate, and nothing will make up for it.

The goal is not to divert the child with good things, but to offer support for the child to get through the inevitable deprivation regarding the loss of the family as he or she knew it. It is not necessarily the end of the world, but it is a time to help a child develop resiliency, rather than to force happiness, in the face of life's bad circumstances that are out of the child's control.

With the exception of early infancy, loving our children does not equate with shielding them from all suffering and providing them with never-ending happiness. Bonds of love are more sturdily built by our attempts to regulate the degree of heartache our children must endure at a level they can handle and by imparting to them the coping skills to face adversity when it comes their way.

Parents' struggles to find the middle ground between gratification and deprivation become exquisitely evident in their difficulties keeping their children out of their bed at night. It is not just where a child sleeps, but also how we put them to bed that highlights the arc of tension between the two poles. A colleague of mine, a well-respected child clinician and researcher of parent–infant relationships, describes to me with great joy his life with his five-month-old baby. He admits, with some guilt, that he or his wife holds their baby until she falls asleep each night, even though all the books are clear that this is a mistake that begins a very bad habit almost impossible to break later. Yet it doesn't feel right to him or his wife just to plop their child into her crib each night. So he and his wife are going to do it their way—gratify their baby and keep her happy by holding her. From their standpoint, to put her to bed to cry it out would both frustrate and deprive her and make them feel like mean parents. But the very fact that my colleague was so eager to share this with me reveals his underlying anxiety—maybe this really is too gratifying and he is thus depriving his daughter of some other developmental achievement, one built on discomfort and coping, rather than happiness and fulfillment. Or maybe he is creating a future hell for him and his wife in the face of a child with an unbreakable "bad habit."

We all know the canned movie plot of the wealthy, overindulged child with mansion, servants, horses in the stable, but no parents available to love or attend to their son or daughter. Full of riches, empty of love. Increasing concern has surfaced that this plot has left the movie screen and is now the plight of the average middle-class

American child. Although an overstatement, I do think the material indulgence of middle-class children today can be understood as another indicator of the tension between gratification and deprivation, where one becomes the other. Showering the children with goods can serve as a bargaining chip in love, in which parents gratify what they think is their child's every whim in order to say, "I love you and I hope you love me." The paradoxical consequence, however, is that they end up leaving the child deprived of the experience of wanting something and of the security of knowing we love them whether a room is filled with toys or not.

We could say the tension between gratification and deprivation is an element of dialectics where something transforms into its opposite. We see it in the wall-to-wall approach to parenting. Our impulse at the end of the day is to gratify all our children's requests and desires to compensate for all they have been deprived of in our absence. We assume that by doing so we are *giving* to our children, until we hear from them one day, "Could you both lay off? I have no breathing space around here."

In this scenario, the mornings have an entirely different flavor, as fairy godparents transform into drill sergeants and the child may well be pushed to the limit of his or her capacities to put things in order, avoid dallying, and handle a myriad of responsibilities to get everybody's day going. After overgratification the night before, the child is now deprived of a sane, slower morning pace, which is compensated for again in the evening by the next round of wall-to-wall parenting and "quality time." And so the parents swing the pendulum from gratification to deprivation and back to gratification, creating a blur between the two.

It is easy to see how the morning deprivation equates with underattention to our children's needs. But so does the evening overinvolvement. We underattend to the messages from our own children. They can be very direct, as when they tell you to lay off. Message: Hovering is smothering. But they can also speak in tongues that need to be deciphered, as when the overindulged child says, "I don't want that anymore," after every granted wish. Translation: "That's not the bucket that needs to be filled. None of this will make me happy because it's really something else I want from you, like telling me, 'No, you can't have everything you want,' or 'Maybe it's not the doll you want but a telephone call from your daddy or a little extra time with me.' " Bells should go off in any situation where you feel you are giving so much but your child is resistant to receiving your gifts. Your child may well be signaling to you to stop overgratifying and start attending to other of his or her needs.

The kinderdult is the personified embodiment of the confusion between gratification and deprivation. We believe the cherub side of the kinderdult to be in need of continual gratification; we think the miniature adult can handle at least a modicum of deprivation, as when we accept what is tolerable rather than what is optimal for them or when we know, deep in our hearts, that we are doing too little when away. So it is no wonder that parents today are in such a quandary about the issue of gratification versus deprivation. They don't even know which is which, there is no easy formula for the balance between the two, and they have no clear vision of who their children are, cherubs to be indulged or miniature adults to be demanded of.

TO LOVE OR TO OBEY

A woman in her sixties sat in my office remembering the death of her mother in the 1930s, when my patient was just a toddler. She recounts that she and her older sister, age four at the time, woke up one morning to find their mother's bed empty. Her older sister recalls running to her father and demanding, "Where's Mommy?" Only then did their father attend to the empty bed and to his children by explaining that Mommy had gone to heaven. Not another word was spoken about it. Some fifty years later, this same older sister writes to my patient about this event, "Remember, in those days children did not ask questions of their parents. They were adults and the children accepted what they were told."

Today, such handling of a mother's death would be considered poor parenting at best, negligence at worst. Children are to be included in family affairs and answered truthfully and respectfully.

We want our children to be autonomous and self-sufficient, rather than compliant or obedient. We must talk to them and also be prepared to listen. We perceive our children as having something to say. We want them to have input into their own lives. We believe that, as a result, we are better parents than our own, more affectionate and understanding, less harsh and rigid.[8]

There is a great deal of merit in this attitude of respect and acknowledgment of our children. We see it as far better than in the "olden days," when children were denied dignity and were subject to their parents' total control. If done with good judgment and in moderation, scaled to the developmental readiness of our child, this shift toward respecting and listening to our children opens the avenues to understanding what our children are really trying to tell us and bolsters our children's confidence that they matter to someone and will be attended to. Daniel Goleman, columnist for *The New York Times,* offers advice to parents about listening: "For the parent who wants to understand better what might be troubling a child, researchers recommend making a specific effort to let the child be heard, something many parents do not take the time to do."[9] Parents are asked to be "active listeners" with their children and take seriously what their children are saying to them, rather than just lecturing them.

In itself, this is very sound advice. But in the hands of overly anxious parents struggling so intensely to win the favor of their children, it can be misused. The advice feeds right into the new bartering for love, either by being taken all too seriously or reinforcing an "overlistening" that is already in place. The advice, when carried to extremes, can overstimulate children's sense of omnipotence and entitlement and create tyrants rather than respected and confident subjects.

Middle-class parents today are at risk for "listening to the children" as if they weren't children at all. In swinging toward the miniature adult pole of the kinderdult concept, they can err in ascribing to their children a sense of rationality and decision-making abilities that are sometimes questionable, if not outlandish. In the words of one mother, "I've treated Alexis as if she had a mind of her own ever since she was a baby. When she was 6 months old and sitting in her crib, I used to ask her what she wanted to do next, what she wanted to eat or to wear."[10]

In their quest for democracy, parents can easily lose sight of the cognitive limits of their child. Sometimes they might overreason with their child. Others times they may hold totally unrealistic expectations of what their child can possibly understand. Alexis's mother probably knows full well that her six-month-old is not going to look up and say, "I'll have Cheerios this morning." But by the time Alexis is a preschooler, her mother may catch herself going on and on explaining why they are not going to have Cheerios for their Thanksgiving feast to a child who has neither the language resources nor the required attention span to absorb an extensive monologue. By school age, rather than loving her mother more for her thoughtful explanations, Alexis may simply look up and say, "Mom, could you just get to the point?"

We need to check our tendency to assault our children with words and explanations. Over and over I find myself sending a message to parents, "Keep it short and sweet." Margot's parents came to see me because her teacher had begun to worry that six-year-old little Margot might be partially deaf, as she appeared to be missing a good deal of what the teacher was saying. A hearing test indicated Margot's hearing was perfect. So what was the problem? I went to observe Margot in her classroom. What I saw was that Margot "tuned out" as soon as the teacher delivered more than a one-sentence communication. In contrast, she heard everything her little friends said to her, no matter how long the message.

I took a family history. I found out that Chris and Michelle, Margot's parents, had promised themselves they would never treat their little girl like they had been treated—Do it because I said so. They had staunchly held to the belief that not only should they listen very carefully to what their child had to say to them, they also owed Margot a full answer to all her questions and a full explanation of all their actions, so that she would never feel things were just being done to her. This meant there was a lot of talking going on in their house, early in the morning and late at night. I observed Margot with her parents and quickly saw that all this talking had become entirely too much for Margot. She had learned to cope with the barrage of words by shutting down, taking in the maximum of what she felt she could handle, which was about one sentence. Chris and Michelle were so caught up in earnestly and lovingly articulating to Margot what they were thinking and feeling that they failed to notice Margot's glazed eyes and blank face. I told them what I think is true for most middle-class parents today: "You talk too much." I advised them to cut down their communications to Margot to a maximum of two sentences at a time, and to pay more attention to the specific messages Margot was sending them and less attention to listening to themselves be benevolent and respectful parents. They tried this and predictably, in due time, as the volume of words dropped markedly at home, Margot's "deafness" was cured.

Parents bend over backwards to take their children seriously, all in the name of love and respect, but more accurately within the spirit of bartering for love. It is here that we can view most poignantly the breakdown of boundaries between parent and child. Rather than wall-to-wall parenting, it is parenting without walls. Instead of generational lines, we now have families-in-the-round. It appears as if everyone has an equal say-so and that hierarchy is obsolete or politically incorrect. Children have not just voting power but veto power in family decisions. Occasionally, sons and daughters even offer their parents advice about what job to take or how to handle their financial affairs. Many children now call parents by their first name. This too is part of the new ultra democracy among middle-class families in which children should be seen, heard, and answered, just like any other adult.

By transforming their child into a friend rather than a dependent, parents hope not just that their child will grow up to be the most creative person he or she can be, but that their child will appreciate how understanding and supportive they are and love them forever and beyond question. Only thus do they believe that they will lose neither the love of the object nor the object itself.

A better solution is to remind ourselves that children are not just short adults. They *are,* as our tax forms remind us, dependents. They rely heavily on hierarchy and generational difference to know that there is a protective rim around them. If we can remember that our children want not just respect, but also safety—from their own impulses, from their own destructiveness, from their own unbridled desires—we take a giant step in extricating ourselves from bartering for love. Children need to be encouraged to assert themselves, but also to establish concern for and recognition of others. They turn to us to get both. Keeping the parent–child boundaries clear is a much better insurance policy than ultra democracy for instilling the balance of assertion and recognition in our children and for letting our children know how deeply we love them.

THE CHILD WE WANT TO LOVE US

Some years ago my husband and I walked to a local cafe late one night to have coffee. We entered a crowded, smoky scene where the majority of the people were in their thirties or forties. My eye was caught by a small child, about three years old, dancing around in the entrance way, dashing in and out. My first thought was, "Rather young to be out so late." His mother was standing in the doorway, chatting with a friend. The little boy grew more and more animated, or perhaps agitated, exuberant but also a bit overwound. Finally it came time for him and his mother to go. His mother approached him, he threw her a challenging look then sprinted toward the back of the cafe, into a swarm of people. With a watchful eye, his mother let him be for a long period of time, time enough for him to bump into several customers and dart recklessly between their legs. He was creating a bit of a commotion, but he was happy.

Now it was really time for them to go. As his mother came toward him, his squeals of delight quickly turned to wails of protest. She grabbed for him while he attempted vigorously to escape her. Mom swept him up and swung him onto her hip, in the process ramming right into a man carrying a hot cup of coffee. Watching the scene, I gasped, while the man cringed and deftly backed up out of harm's way. The mother took no notice at all. She sailed out of the restaurant, she and her pal for the night gone for the evening.

In the process of watching this unfold, I made eye contact with the man holding the simmering cup of coffee. He shook his head in disgust and muttered irately to the mother's back, "He should be in bed where he belongs." And I must admit, I sympathized with him. This child was being granted far too much freedom and autonomy for his own good in an environment where running through people's legs and kicking and flailing (normal for a child) was totally inappropriate, if not dangerous. At the same time I felt guilty for "blaming" the mother. Knowing nothing of her circumstances, I ran through a series of thoughts, "Perhaps she has no child care and this is her only way to get out. Maybe she has a work shift that dictates late night outings with her child to get to see him. Compared to my parents' generation, how nice to give him spontaneity and a fun time at the cafe. What an adventure this would have been for me if I had been allowed to do that as a child." But then I recalled the near spill of the steaming coffee, the man and his look of anger, and my own desire to have a late night excursion away from the world of children. I reflected on this mother's total indulgence of her son until it was truly time to leave. Although she was effective in setting a final limit, I wondered whether she was also caught up in bartering for love.

I learned from my own waffling reactions how temporarily confused I was about the new bartering for love, and how confused most other people must be alongside me. I came to the conclusion that it is good that we have made more room for our children amidst the world of adults than when I was a child, but that we have gone overboard in the latitude we have given them to "run the show." It is nothing but a burden for our children when we bid so strongly for their love and fear so greatly that we will lose it.

Parents go overboard to give their child autonomy and respect. A family comes to me for help because their ten-year-old daughter, Ashley, has developed separation anxieties and refuses to be apart from her parents except when she attends school. Before this, she had managed separations just fine. The parents have not gone out by themselves in over a year. They are at their wits' end, but at the same time do not want to push Ashley into doing something that would traumatize her. Indeed, she has cried and wailed whenever they have tried to leave her, even with her grandparents with whom she had always stayed in the past. Further, she will hardly let her parents finish a conversation without literally stepping right between them.

When I interview Ashley, she vacillates between precocious self-confidence and sophistication and regressive anxiety and whininess. I take her seriously when she tells me how scared she is when her mother or father are not with her, but I also make note of her resistance and anger when I suggest that we could help her with this so that she could again enjoy time away from her parents. I know from the history Ashley's parents gave me that they had spent a year in Asia during which time her parents never left her side, except when she went to school. It was only upon their return that the present symptoms surfaced. Prior to their trip she had been on a healthy track toward independence.

In discussing with Ashley why she had developed such fears of being without her parents, I probed different possibilities: the loss of their house in a fire, the fear of getting older and going through puberty, worries about her parents' relationship. Each time she adamantly shook her head, "No," and explained that it just didn't feel like that. Then I suggested that perhaps it was hard to give up a good thing—the unending attention from her parents during that year abroad. She readily nodded her head in agreement. She knew perfectly well what was going on, but in no way could she get herself to stop.

I began to recognize the protection racket that had emerged in this family. Ashley had been derailed in her forward development by the year of "great indulgence." She was going to make her parents pay for it by keeping them under her thumb, never more than a stone's throw away. She knew she had to go to school, and couldn't balk at that, but the rest of her life was more "voluntary." In bartering for love, she could make her parents stay by her side out of fear that they would harm her if they didn't and worry that she would be extremely angry at them if they left her.

There is a happy ending to the story, but it took my therapeutic intervention to recommend that separations be reinstituted gradually, with tools to help Ashley deal with them (phone calls home to check in and "transitional objects," such as notes from her parents, to remind her of their love and to give her comfort) and confidence conveyed to her that she, in fact, had the resources to negotiate brief separations. With both Ashley and her parents caught up in bartering for love and her parents listening so seriously to her "I can't, too scary" messages, Ashley had been gratified in her immediate wishes but deprived of the opportunity to get on with the tasks of middle childhood, which include experiencing brief or even more extended separations from family and home. Paradoxically, Ashley's parents' attempts to respect her autonomy ended up impeding it.

To put it another way, the child in bartering for love is at risk for the syndrome of "false independence." Children like to play house and be grown ups, but it is only play. If we take such play too seriously, we put them in the driver's seat well before they are ready.

Although we think we are catering to our children in acceding to their wishes and demands, we are pushing them beyond their limits to assume independence in life. Putting our children on a par with ourselves and bending over backward to acknowledge their individuality and demonstrate we are not thwarting them has the untoward consequence of taking their childhood away. If, instead, we probe more deeply into what they are communicating below the surface and what they really need from us, we can hear them asking just to be little children who can count on their elders to place reasonable demands on them to help bring them forward, but not too fast.

In extreme cases, a child can crack under the pressure of the two tenets of bartering for love. A colleague of mine was asked to do a psychological evaluation of a teenager. The girl had suddenly announced that she was not going to school anymore and had been home for about two weeks. My colleague came to me for a consultation. I suggested that she ask the parents how they had come to the decision to let her stay home. My colleague followed my suggestion, and called to report the following response. First, the parents looked at her with an expression of total shock and confusion. And then, they readily offered, "Why, she makes all her own decisions. We haven't made a decision for her since she was two years old, and even then we're not sure that was right."

Here is what this teenage girl had to say to my colleague about that. "All my life in my family I've been feeling like I wear a mask everyday. Every night I show up with my mask on."[11] How could she feel like herself when her parents failed to recognize that she was just a child who needed some help and guidance, not a miniature adult ready to determine her own life? Her well-meaning but confused mother and father intended to be good parents by respecting her autonomy and giving her freedom. In bartering for love, they hoped this would strengthen their bonds with her, but instead it led to a psychiatric crisis in adolescence. She had been deprived of a sense of authenticity and instead felt that her life with her parents had been an ongoing charade. All this might have been avoided if her parents had done something as simple as making decisions for her until she was ready to make them for herself and checking to make sure there was a good balance between autonomy and parent directives appropriate to the girl's age as she grew.

Another colleague brought to my child consultation group an almost identical story. She is working with a twelve-year-old girl who is manifesting separation anxiety and school refusal. The parents are divorced. The father balks at telling his daughter to do anything: "It's not my style. I never tell people what to do." The daughter is allowed to decide whether or not to see her father, whether or not to stay in her present school, and whether or not to come to therapy. When the therapist recommends to the father that the adults, not the children, should set the schedule for visitation, he lamely agrees, but then asserts that he does not like to impose things on his child.

My colleague describes Jeanette, her twelve-year-old patient as a "false little adult." She reports that Jeanette's father, in an effort to be "Mr. Nice Guy," relates to both his children as "miniature adults," not as children who need structure and guidance. In response, Jeanette has become imperious and demanding, expecting the world to revolve around her needs and wishes. My colleague's assessment: "Jeanette is the kid who is like this little adult on the outside and mush on the inside."[12]

Her work has been to get the father to *like* to impose things on his child and to recognize that nice guys don't always win when it comes to raising a child who feels healthy and secure. If successful, she may help this child develop sturdiness both on the inside and the outside, with the capacity not only to assert herself, but to show concern for and recognition of others. She may also be able to extricate the father from bartering for love and put him on a path of healthier relationships with his children.

In our continual rush to gratify our children, we often deprive them of taking on responsibilities for themselves or for others. Yet at the same time, our tremendous focus on respect and acknowledgment of our children burdens them with too many responsibilities. The freedoms we allow our children in bartering for love force them to adapt by assuming responsible behaviors that tax their developmental capacities. Children given equal voting power in the family may have to learn decision-making skills before they are cognitively ready. Children allowed to make all their own decisions may be forced to be hypervigilant about their own welfare and best interests at a time when parents would best be handling that function.

In bartering for love we see another push on the pendulum of confused and guilt-ridden parenting, with the child holding on for dear life on the arcs of the swing. Our major work as parents is to challenge our beliefs that our ties to our children are tenuous and our acceptance by them is dependent on keeping them happy and pleased with us. We have unfortunately come to live by the credo that our demands, our foibles, and our inability to shield our children from suffering jeopardize the bonds of love and should be avoided at all costs. However, parents can extricate themselves from love bartering by learning to be more authentic and present with their children, placing demands as well as granting them, garnering respect as well as giving it, and assuaging the parental anxiety that they stand to lose their child's love on a moment's notice. As we adopt these new ways of being, we offer our children a better chance of developing true independence and authentic individuality. We spare them the wild oscillations between gratification and deprivation. And most importantly, we free them from the burden of being the grantors rather than the grantees of love.

CHAPTER EIGHT

• • • • • •

Use the Rod,
Lose the Child

A generation who once raised hell is now raising kids.
—Promotional line for FAMILY LIFE magazine[1]

Love and anger is the parental dilemma. Amazing enough, even though all loving parents get angry and furious and rage at their kids, not many people talk about it.
—BARBARA SAMALIN[2]

If a generation who once raised hell is now raising children, how do they discipline these children? The answer is, with a great deal of difficulty. Setting limits and enforcing discipline are tasks fraught with great anxiety for today's parents. If there is one place parents flounder, it is here. They tend to go overboard in one direction or the other. Most notable is the inability of many parents to *just say no.* With great trepidation, some parents consider even raising their voices a violent response, whereas others lose control completely and contribute to the rise in reported incidents of child abuse. And on either end of the spectrum, nobody wants to talk about it. Appropriate modulation and incorporation of healthy aggression into parenting is completely off kilter among mothers and fathers today. And it has almost become a taboo subject.

We have already learned that in bartering for love, parents want to be pals not enforcers to their children. Further, love, rather than obedience, has become the guiding principle in parent–child relationships. The dilemmas of discipline are just a subset of the larger problem of love bartering. But the dimensions and ramifications of this subset are so monumental as to warrant a separate discussion. In the historical shift from obedience to love and from authoritarian to democratic modes of child rearing, what becomes of limit setting, sanctions for poor behavior, and boundaries of acceptable behavior?

The answer is simple, but the explanations complex. "Spare the rod, spoil the child" has been radically transformed to "Use the rod, lose the child." Raise a hand or even a voice to your child and stand to fail miserably as a parent and destroy your child in the process. This is the new belief system. To understand the meaning behind "use the rod, lose the child," we have to look at parents' and the entire culture's ambivalence about aggression, parents' fear of authority, their beliefs about the damage that misuse or even use of authority and aggression can inflict on a child, and mothers' and fathers' actual struggles over limit setting and disciplinary actions.

NO HITTING

Francine, a mother of a three-year-old, is sitting across from me in my consulting room, wringing her hands. Tears are streaming down her face. She has come to discuss the posttraumatic stress reaction in her daughter, Colette, following a physical injury. But in the course of our hour together she tells me, with great shame, that she may have further traumatized her child. How? Her child darted toward the street, and she, fearing another accident, slapped her child's hand to stop her. Parents are not supposed to strike their children, and she had transgressed—transgressed by performing an age-old human act of protection of the young: In face of danger, with no time for words, use your body.

These days we do not like to think of ourselves as so primitive as to strike out physically at a child. If we should do so, we are flooded with guilt that we have been brutal or abusive. In most states, there are even laws to prohibit such actions. But a child has neither the reasoning powers nor the internal controls that would allow us *in all instances* to avoid using our bodies when words will not work or are not quickly enough available. So occasionally we do. In a psychologically minded society that attributes irreparable harm to early trauma, we are then further plagued by the guilt that the harm of inflicted blows to our children is not just temporary but permanent.

I am not advocating spanking or physical punishment as an optimal disciplining tactic. But we need to ask ourselves why we have become so up in arms about an occasional tap on the wrist or swat on the bottom. I myself was a child lightly spanked by my mother once in a while to put an end to my morning tantrums. It worked. I calmed down and got on with my day. I seem none the worse for wear. Nevertheless, many years later, I too became one of those parents who never spanked.

Our intense negative reactions to hitting are emblematic of a broader phenomenon: In the era of permissive and democratic child rearing, parental anger finds no legitimate place. This has become a central problem of parenting today. Directives to parents in the face of conflict with their children involve staying calm and reasonable in all events, even when up against the most outrageous or dangerous behaviors from their sons or daughters. As for their own anger, parents are to keep it in check.

This new sensibility about parental anger is best exemplified in the immensely popular Parent Effectiveness Training that originated in the 1970s. In books and classes throughout the country, parents were taught the art of "active listening" with their children. They were instructed by Dr. Thomas Gordon and his followers that their own experience of anger in response to their children was not really what they were feeling. Anger was just a secondary feeling used by the parent to blame, punish, or teach a child a lesson. People just make themselves angry when deep inside they are feeling something else because of what their child has done.

Parents are instructed to get in touch with their primary feelings, such as disappointment, hurt, or worry, and purge themselves of anger in their interactions with their children. This will prepare them for the proper attitude in attending to their children, one that is both receptive and active but never emotionally out of control. Parents are encouraged to trust their children's capacity to handle feelings and work through them, to appreciate that feelings are transitory not permanent, and lastly, to recognize their children as unique people separate from their parents.[3]

Even with the emphasis on exploring children's feelings with them, parents themselves are to remain rational. Emotions are to be *talked about* ("It makes me upset when you do that, Sammy"), but not demonstrated in the raw—neither in words nor in actions. It's a little like asking parents to be saints.

Civilized, reasoning parents are not to fly off the handle. But civilized, reasoning parents are also having a difficult time managing their own feelings of aggression, feelings which I believe are part and parcel of the child rearing process and are particularly aggravated in an era that gives all the responsibility but no support to parents to raise their children adequately. It is a rare parent who does not in a stressful moment fantasize, either consciously or unconsciously, about the possibilities of infanticide. I am reminded of my mother, never a follower of permissive parenting. Her common refrain "I'll kill you," following one of our transgressions, was never taken seriously by me or my brothers, nor did it ever seem to consume her with guilt. Yet I myself would choke on the words before ever invoking them with my own children. Why have I not adopted my mother's refrain?

I am not as free as my mother to express aggression. I fear very much that words can hurt. I censor my angry feelings before I let them loose on my children. I am a product of a different generation, the youth growing up in the 1960s committed to eliminating the generation gap through permissiveness, openness, and understanding. Telling my children "I'll kill you" would be antithetical to that goal. I used to be confident of the superior wisdom of my actions, but now I wonder. Perhaps there is something to be learned from the freedom with which my mother was able to call out her seemingly murderous fantasies.

Wondering is not just an academic question for me. My struggles with my own children, particularly my first, forced me to confront the reality that my children needed less protection from my anger than I was providing. I believe that for many years my oldest child suffered from too much understanding and not enough guidance. I began asking myself, "What would be so terrible if Rebecca knew how angry I was right now?" The more freedom I felt to express my disapproval or anger, in a respectful way, the better our relationship became and the better Rebecca did.

I am not the only parent who has been confused. Recently I asked parents in a workshop addressing parenting as the "impossible profession" to name an incident in which they felt inadequate in an interchange with their child. I was swamped with a set of responses in which a singular worry surfaced: "I'm not good at disciplining my child" / "I don't know what to do with my angry feelings." The following mother's response was emblematic:

> My daughter is 3½. She will continue to do something such as bother her sibling after I have asked her to stop, yelled for her to stop, threatened with a time out, etc. So I put her in her room for 5 minutes, but she won't stay in her room, she keeps coming back out. So then—after escorting her back several times, I spank her once on her bottom. She cries and I feel guilty, I don't believe in spanking, and I can't figure out how the situation deteriorated so far. I end up feeling like I am the *worst parent* and that I have *ruined my child* and she will be affected for the rest of her life [italics added].

Many themes run through this story: a mother's difficulty in managing her daughter, a child who does not take no for an answer, a parent experiencing herself becoming out of control and violent, the child's wailing response, the subsequent wounding of the mother's parenting confidence and her worry that she has damaged her child for life. Like Francine, who cried because she slapped her child to prevent her from running into the street, the central dynamic looming large for this mother and the great majority of parents today is their difficulty in living with their own aggressive impulses and their lack of confidence in integrating aggressive or angry feelings into appropriate discipline of their children. I can attest to the prevalence of their struggle by the number of times I find myself consulting with parents who are operating from either one extreme or the other—too much or too harsh discipline; too little or too ineffectual discipline. It is not often that I find someone who falls right in the middle.

The consultation work is always the same. First, I explore with the parents their expectations for their children. Are they reasonable? The overdiscipliner often expects too much, the underdiscipliner too little. Then we explore the parents' anger or disapproval—is it reasonable in response to the situation at hand? Again, the overdiscipliner's anger or reaction is often overblown, the underdiscipliner's disturbingly nonexistent. After attempting to gauge the level of feeling or reaction to match the child's actions appropriately, the last step is to explore ways of expressing the anger or disapproval that are neither frightening nor harmful to the child but help contain and control behaviors that the child is not able to control on his or her own. In this way, we get to the middle ground.

We have to look at the society around us, the childhood behind us, and the psyche within us to understand why so many people need such help in modulating aggression. Let us begin with the society. We have entered an era of permissiveness in which the scales are tipped toward gratification over deprivation. However, the era of permissiveness in no way equates with permission to express aggression, only permission to capitalize on love. As Christopher Lasch explained in *The Culture of Narcissism*: "The new permissiveness extends largely to expression of libidinal instincts, not to aggression. A bureaucratic society that stresses cooperation, interpersonal give and take, cannot allow many legitimate outlets of anger. Even in the family, which is supposed to allow expression to feelings denied expression elsewhere, anger threatens the precarious equilibrium that members of the family try so hard to preserve."[4]

We just want everyone to be happy. Aggression is not considered a happy emotion, nor is it considered a productive sentiment. And yet the statistics on violence go up every year. If we zero in on parenting today, it seems paradoxical that so much emphasis should be put on the inhibition of aggression in parent–child interactions while the degree of child abuse in this country remains alarmingly high. There is certainly a rift between philosophy and practice, and the extreme contrast between the two highlights the difficulty we are having with the issue of aggression and parenting. Is it the practice or the philosophy that is off balance, or both?

During the birth of this country, in the Puritan era, corporal, even capital punishment of children was condoned. Today the public stance is "no hitting." While visiting Chicago recently, I came across an article about a woman who was charged but not convicted of child abuse for hitting her child in public. A visitor from the Pilgrim era would be astounded. But now it is considered a possible crime to discipline your child with your hand. If we translate such an act as a form of aggression in parenting, we can say that parental aggression is in violation of, rather than in accordance with public philosophy and policy.

Public policy certainly feeds into parents' hesitance and ambivalence about expressing anger toward their children. In California it is public law that any health professional or educator who *suspects* child abuse inflicted on a child with whom they come in contact must make a report to either the police or the child protection service. Recently, the child protection unit knocked on the door of a family in Berkeley. Their daughter attended an exclusive private school in the area. Her teacher had noticed suspicious red marks on her neck. She felt obligated to report them to the Child Protection Service for investigation of abuse. A social worker was sent out to investigate. The parents, not very receptive to the intrusion, explained that the marks were a permanent birthmark. The social worker was not convinced. The parents, in their frustration, became more belligerent. The social worker became more suspicious. She threatened to remove all the children from the home and place them in emergency foster care. Medical documentation of the birth mark was provided, the case was cleared up, and the family resumed their life as normal—except they will never forget that knock at the door and what could have transpired had they not cleared their name.

A mother tells her story to *Newsweek*. Her twelve-year-old daughter, Kelly, went to a friend's house and reported to her friend's mother that her stepfather had hit her. That mother called the school. The school counselor called Kelly in that day for an interview. By that time Kelly had embellished her story to, "He always hits me." The school counselor called the sheriff's department and social services. The child was taken into custody and the parents investigated. The mother was told by the deputy sheriff, "Your daughter is fine. I have her with me. And she has reported your husband for child abuse. Extreme and ongoing." By the mother's report, Kelly's stepfather had given her three whacks on the behind that morning for not cleaning her mess. The mother explains, "This is a parent's prerogative. He'd done nothing wrong or illegal. My husband is not abusive. He stepped into my life nine years ago. He chose to help me raise my three children and has done so with love. I'm not saying he is perfect, but who is?" The deputy sheriff interviewed the girl and determined that no abuse had occurred and that the child had stretched her story.[5] But in an age of "no hitting," her stepfather could have ended up in jail. And the public stigma attached to these parents as suspected abusers may be irreversible.

A set of policies established to protect children ironically provides at the same time the potential for a witch hunt, such that parents live in fear that any discipline may be perceived by some authority as abuse. Although some parents are indeed out of control and out of line in disciplining their children, the great majority of parents are left to question whether *any* aggressive impulse, when expressed, is abusive. Spanking and hitting may be antithetical to respectful relationships with our children, but the baby gets thrown out with the bath water when we begin to doubt whether *any* form of firm action is valid. In a society that appears to be becoming increasingly violent or out of control in its modulation of aggression, it is fascinating to notice how much parents are now policed on their levels of aggressiveness. Bang bang, but no hitting.

AFRAID OF OUR OWN SHADOW

Now let us turn to the childhood behind us and the psyche within us. Parenthood starts while we are still children when we first develop the essential human skills for interactions with others and begin to integrate the basic components of our personality. To do this, love and aggression are two major forces to contend with. Through libido (erotic impulses), we develop the capacity to seek pleasure, to attach to others, and to care for both ourselves and others. Through aggression, we establish boundaries between ourselves and others and strengthen our life force. In health, we are able to integrate both our erotic and aggressive components.

The erotic part seems straightforward, the aggression part more mysterious. An infant appears to be born with a life force that gets stimulated by an experience of opposition, the first one being the actual exit from the birth canal. These experiences of opposition (as simple as to-and-fro or rocking movements) bring along the development of the aggressive impulse. In this sense, early aggression almost equates with activity (the fetus kicking in the womb, the infant nibbling at the breast). It is not destructive and is not aimed to hurt.

To achieve satisfaction of the aggressive impulse requires some experience of "butting up" against something. This is not so for the "love" impulses, which can derive satisfaction within an experience of merging or fusion. It is the aggressive impulse that drives the infant to search for an environment, a "not-me" that is distinguished from a "me." In a social environment that is good but not always perfect, the infant increasingly grows to learn that a world exists outside itself that will sometimes be frustrating and never totally identical to the infant itself, leading to anger on the part of the infant. This translates to a parent who is there, but gradually over time is not able to nor should grant the baby's every desire or wish as it comes up. It also translates into a parent who will be stably there and not be retaliatory or decimated in the face of the infant's own aggressive impulses. Here is an opposition that facilitates the firm development of a sense of self that stops here and a sense of another person that begins there, the me and the not-me.

Three parts of the human personality may evolve to negotiate love and aggression: (1) a true self, with me and not-me firmly established, and with some fusion of the aggressive and erotic elements; (2) a self governed by erotic experiences, which robs the individual of a sense of external reality; or (3) a self ruthlessly given over to aggression, where being real is felt only in being in opposition to another. The true self is the goal of healthy development, where the fusion of aggressive and erotic components of an experience make it all the more real and vibrant.[6] In other words, love and aggression go together like a horse and carriage. We can all capture the significance of this if we consider the phenomenon of lovemaking, in which the fusion of our tender feelings toward our partner with some mutual feeling of opposition, otherness, or assertiveness can make for the most intense, satisfying, and real of experiences.

In these terms, aggressiveness is not inherently destructive; it only becomes so later in development when it is attached to an object that is hated or feared or when its intent is to hurt or to destroy. In its most generic form, aggression is the means by which we create separateness between ourselves and another person. So why are so many American parents afraid of it or having such a hard time integrating it with love?

Recall that beginning in the post-World War II era many of us were brought up by the bible of Benjamin Spock, believed to have a silver spoon in our mouths, and destined to live as if the world was our oyster. With the new overemphasis on gratification, we may very well have been robbed of opportunities to feel the opposition that creates boundaries between ourselves and those who were our elders. The permissiveness toward pleasuring-seeking activities but squelching of aggression in many families may have resulted in a repression of personal aggressiveness in individuals. The great majority of us may have been left stranded in the second style of personality, where erotic impulses govern our feelings and behaviors but rob us of that "intimate edge"[7] between self and other. These become the parents who have difficulty even raising their voices with their children. For others of us, less fortunate, the derailing of the development of healthy aggressiveness may paradoxically have culminated in a compensatory overly aggressive personality, the third type, in which frustration and anger cannot be checked by feelings of love, and life becomes an experience of "kill or be killed." These are the parents who lose control and harm their children with destructive feelings and behaviors.

There has been much discussion of the abusive, overly aggressive parent, but virtually no attention paid to the inhibited, underaggressive parent governed by guilt and anxiety. The latter group, I believe, represents a vast number of parents today, both mothers and fathers. I am talking about the parents who are truly afraid of their own shadow, the shadow being their own aggressive impulses that, in good health, would naturally come to bear in raising children. How interesting that we have a society that carefully monitors overaggressive parents, but overlooks the underaggressive parents who are reeking havoc on both themselves and their children. It is about time that we direct our focus to this phenomenon. Forty years ago, D. W. Winnicott had already alerted us to the problem: "If society is in danger, it is not because of man's aggressiveness but because of the repression of personal aggressiveness in individuals."[8] That childhood legacy of repression of aggression is precisely what makes parenting so perilous for so many, and to which I want to devote the remainder of this discussion.

A couple comes to consult with me about their four-year-old child, Benjamin, who has outbursts any time his parents tell him to do something or tell him he cannot do something he wanted to do. Maxine and Tom Jackson are a lovely couple, soft spoken, thoughtful, and very open. Tom explains how he had spent the day with Benjamin and Benjamin had pulled out all the stops. Father felt helpless to stop the onslaught of taunts and rebellious acts on Benjamin's part. They just kept coming. The house was in a shambles. Tom reports, with great chagrin, that he finally "lost it" and yelled at his son, telling him in a loud voice to stop it, after Benjamin began throwing hard objects at his bedroom door after being asked to take a time out. The father feels terribly ashamed and guilty about his yelling. I ask him what effect the so-called yelling had. He responds that the child indeed calmed down and stopped acting out.

For both parents I have to redefine father's behavior. It is not an act of brutality. In the future, Tom might train himself to respond earlier, before he is ready to explode, and substitute "firm voice and demeanor" for loud yelling. But in the meantime, Tom's raised voice in that moment served as a clear signal to Benjamin that his father really meant business, a signal that up to that point Tom was having tremendous difficulty putting out. Yelling may not be an effective mode of parenting, but communicating that you mean business is. Tom also needed to be reassured that every parent, if truly human, will lose his or her temper from time to time and raise his or her voice. It is only a serious problem when the raised voice unduly frightens the child, becomes chronic, or signifies that parent as well as child are out of control.

Maxine then reports that the day after Dad's day from hell with his son, Benjamin said to her, "Daddy's mad, he had a mad face yesterday." Mom reassured Benjamin that sometimes Daddy might get mad, but that really didn't mean anything and that he still loved Benjamin. I suggest that mother might try another strategy, so as to make sense of cause and effect for Benjamin. She can explain to Benjamin that yes, Daddy or anybody else might get mad when Benjamin dumped all the clean laundry all over the floor or some such thing, and that they are going to help Benjamin so that he might not do so many things that could get other people mad. Maxine stares at me in amazement: "You mean I could do that? I always thought that telling your kid that if they were mean, nobody would like them was a really terrible thing and you could damage them for life." I respond that yes, such a message could be damaging, but that isn't what I am suggesting. The character assassination she was imagining is very different from communicating to your child that certain of his behaviors get other people angry. She sighs and says, "You know, we just don't know how to do this. We've never been around kids before and this is our first, so we just don't know." And my heart goes out to Maxine and Tom as I think, "And it's also your terrible fears of your own aggressiveness that leave you both tied in knots or exploding like a volcano after holding your anger in for so long."

Maxine also tells me in this consultation that she has read the book *The Difficult Child*. She has learned from it that we must be understanding about temperament, but firm about behaviors. Maxine recognizes that her child is wired in a certain way that makes him more eruptive and sensitive to overstimulation. Therefore, she thinks she must express only understanding to Benjamin. She has not gotten it that the behaviors that emanate from that temperamental style still need some shaping and alteration if Benjamin is going to make a go of it in the world. I introduce the concept of firm understanding. Maxine appears extremely relieved and hungry for the help. For the first time, somebody is giving her permission to express the anger she is constantly working to suppress and even to bring to the surface the deeper feelings of personal aggressiveness that have been repressed since childhood for fear of the harm they could do to herself or others. Moreover, the permission comes with the promise of no damage to their child.

Maxine and Tom Johnson will make it out of the woods. They are motivated and caring parents. But they have been terrified of destroying their child through their own aggressive acts and confused by the very moments when they were able to fuse love and aggression effectively and do the right thing, that is, let Benjamin know they meant business.

So inhibited in their own aggression, they have paradoxically created a child who hits and punches them and knows no bounds to his own. (As a footnote, it is remarkable to observe that modern middle-class parents do not allow themselves to hit their children, but they let their children hit *them* all the time.) Benjamin is obsessed with guns and weapons, and will create one from any old scrap he can find. He has chosen as his most provocative behavior lunging for and climbing up to any sharp, dangerous object—knives, scissors, nail clippers. It never dawned on Maxine and Tom to remove such items completely from his reach. This we could certainly understand as an unconscious aggressive act on their part. Benjamin, clever boy that he is, broadcasts the message loud and clear: "We're having trouble with aggression in our family; I have too much, my parents have too little."

A colleague in my child consultation group raised the problem of children who announce they no longer want to be in therapy and parents who support that, despite their child's obvious psychological problems or behavioral difficulties. In further exploration of a particular case, we learned about a mother who had it in her mind to send her child to therapy only if it was going to be pleasurable and make her child feel happy. She described therapy to her daughter as a place to play games and have fun. The problem is that therapy is not always fun, and it sometimes necessitates the uncovering of great unhappiness before things can get better. Sure enough, her daughter was not having fun in her sessions. But she was not having fun out in the world either, where she was failing miserably in making friends and developing relationships. The girl was vitriolic in expressing her hatred toward the therapist, calling her every bad name in her eight-year-old vocabulary. She was never coming back to this hateful place. It was not fun, like her mother had promised. The mother, present at the time, did nothing to stop her daughter in her verbal abuse of the therapist. She also did nothing to stop her daughter when she tore the house apart at home. The therapist took her firmest stance in recommending the need for ongoing therapy and asking for the parents' support in making it be their choice, not their child's, as to whether she would attend therapy. The mother balked. In no way was she going to inflict suffering on her child and make her miserable. That would be mean and abusive.

We do not know in what ways this mother was identified with her daughter and what unconscious resistance she might have had to her daughter being in therapy or actually getting better. What we do know is that her avoidance of any perceived act of aggressiveness toward her child seemed directly correlated with a surfeit of hateful aggression on her child's part. Perhaps the child is acting out the mother's aggression for her. Not unrelated, the child may be unconsciously locked into a desperate struggle to get her mother to express the kind of healthy aggressiveness that necessitates opposition and leads to a clear demarcation between self and other. Without this kind of demarcation, a child rarely succeeds in personal relationships, which was certainly the case for this child. We also know that this mother's aggressiveness was still leaking out despite her disavowal of it, displaced onto the therapist and enacted in her refusal to follow through in getting her child the help she needed. All in the name of that specific transaction in bartering for love in which parental aggression toward a child must be removed to avoid loss or damage.

If the parent is afraid of his or her own aggressive impulses, then the parent will be incapable of fully experiencing a separateness between self and child. The me–not-me world will be impaired, both for parent and for child. And if cultural and personal forces prohibit the parent from achieving at least that much, the parent will have even greater difficulty with the higher level task predicated on the presence of healthy personal aggressiveness—the capacity to become an authority figure for the child.

DOWN WITH BOSSES

A generation raised with the slogan "Smash Authority" is certainly going to have some problems facing parenthood. Parents with an allegiance to their fraying youth status have found that this phrase has not served them well as parents. The belief that Never-Never Land, a world with no parents to tell you when to go to bed, could be extended to themselves *and* their children has simply not worked when facing the reality of an actual child to raise. Recall the mother who began talking to her daughter, Alexis, when she was only six months old, asking her what she would like to wear that day or what she would like for breakfast. There is a sequel to the story. When Alexis turned four, her mother and father found themselves in the position of wanting their child to mind them from time to time. The mother reports the following interchange: "The other day I told her, 'Alexis, you're going to do this right now because I say so!' She looked up at me astounded—as if to say, 'What's going on here? You're changing the rules on me!' " The father gives his version: "For years my wife and I have urged our kids to think for themselves. Now, when we want them to do something we have to appeal to their self-interest, their sense of fairness and logic. I probably use the word 'obey' once every six months. But sometimes it's frustrating when you want them to go along with you."[9]

Alexis's parents are frustrated because they have failed to lay the groundwork for "benevolent authority," by which children by age four would have internalized the expectation that parents indeed run the show and are responsible for shaping and guiding their children's behavior. The treatment of their tiny infant as an autonomous reasoning being actually reveals a false notion of me and not-me. In an authentic establishment of separateness and of external reality, differences, not similarities, between parent and child must be highlighted. When parents cater to the miniature adult pole of the kinderdult axis, merging, rather than individuation, occurs between parent and child. The child is perceived as a little clone of the parent. Along with such merging, in which the component of personal aggressiveness is lacking, comes the repudiation of authority, which requires that one person indeed must establish some sense of differentness, control, and greater wisdom than the other.

Middle-class people bring to the parenting arena permissiveness, openness, understanding, and respect for their children's autonomy. They are then hit with their child's competing need for guidance, direction, and a parent who is *not* just like them. This has forced parents to confront the fact that the real issue for the Peter Pan generation is not the preservation of youth for the sake of their children, but their own unwillingness to leave childhood behind and take on the position of adult authority that is their inevitable legacy in growing up. For the question, "Who are they doing this for, themselves or their children?" the answer is clear: for themselves, all the while genuinely believing it will be best for the children.

Nowhere have we uncovered a healthy child-rearing culture that practices the complete abnegation of adult authority. Even in perfect democracy there is a need for leaders. Today's parents struggle hard to accept the role of authority, which, by dictionary definition, involves "the right to determine, adjudicate, or otherwise settle issues or disputes; the right to control, command or determine."[10]

Even when Dr. Spock himself assures us that "children don't have to be uptight or hostile individuals because of a strict upbringing,"[11] parents are not convinced. Why? Because it is not a matter of convincing. Instead, we have to uncover parents' deeper psychological defenses that inhibit firm upbringing—specifically, the avoidance of the aggressive energy or assertive force that underlies assuming authority. Often the conscious explanation goes something like this: "My parents were very authoritarian, and I vowed I would never do the same with my own children." We want our children to feel respected and free, rather than oppressed and bound. But when we dig deeper, we discover other forces at work, namely, our fear that if we call on that pool of energy from within ourselves, we might harm our children and drive them away. To become an authority quickly equates with being a tyrant, an evil being who will suppress spontaneity and creativity in our children.

It will help us tremendously as parents to undo these aversions to authority. To be an authority figure to our children is to instill in them a respect for our wisdom and a trust in our ability to shepherd them through childhood with their best interests in mind. When fused with love, it allows the child to feel both cared for and protected, while at the same time setting up a "benign opposition" in which a child can test his or her muster by challenging authority, but only within certain limits. It is also a sharing of our deepest selves, communicating to our children our values and beliefs and the things we feel most strongly about. When a parent fails to establish such a relationship with his or her child, the irony is that both parent and child are left with a surfeit of unbridled aggression, the very emotion the underaggressive, authority-aversive parent desperately attempts to steer clear of.

Christopher Lasch gives an account of a father who refuses to punish his rebellious adolescent daughter. The father does not want to give her the satisfaction of a punishment, as he fully recognizes that this is what she is looking for, and he is not willing to fall for the bait. Instead, he gives in to her wishes, avoiding quarrels. Across the board, this father has tried to be a best friend to his children, to be anything but an authoritarian parent. But strangely enough, his children instead experience him as a tyrant. This poor father is totally befuddled. He cannot understand why his son fears that he is going to hit him and his daughter has memories of being beaten as a small child, when he claims that neither event will or ever did happen. Lasch attributes the children's delusional fantasies to the parent's abdication of authority. Rather than such abdication creating a field of safety and acceptance for the child, the child's fear of punishment is only intensified.[12]

The repression of personal aggressiveness on the father's part does not go unnoticed, at least at an unconscious level, by his children. The children respond to the parent's unconscious struggle with aggressive forces. They tune in to the more violent aspects that remain repudiated and repressed. If the parent is afraid to let even a little out, it must truly be something quite horrible. Thus, the children generate overblown fantasies of punishment tied to the exercise of arbitrary, overwhelming violence, a violence that the children unconsciously imagine must be going on inside their father, if he is so frightened to take a position of even mild authority lest he destroy somebody.

Shirking authority only stokes the fires of our children's more primitive fears of raw aggression and violence, and therefore it becomes a very serious problem in child rearing. From the children's (unconscious) perspective, if we parents are so vigilant in checking these emotions and shying away from positions of authority, great danger must be lurking. It may even explain why some children give false reports of child abuse by a parent.

An eight-year-old reports to her teacher that her mother had beaten her badly that morning. The teacher is taken aback, for this mother has always impressed her as such a mild mannered, even meek woman. What actually transpired is that the mother had let the girl run wild that morning while barricading herself in her bedroom in frustration and despair. The child responded not to what her mother *had* done, but what she fantasized her mother *wanted* to do to her that morning. She was not lying, simply imagining.

Within such imagining we also see the children's own anxieties and inabilities to control their own impulses. We don't want our children to fear us. But when we renege on authority, the children are left with no guidelines, external or internal, to keep them in check. They begin to fear that the brake system has failed, that nobody or nothing will stop them from unleashing all of their impulses on the world, a situation that, as they grow, is not welcomed but instead makes them feel out of control.[13] In the accounts above, out-of-control Benjamin, the little girl who said an abusive "No" to therapy, and the son and daughter in the family described by Lasch are all children suffering from such conflicts about impulse control, the unintentional and unexpected result of parents who vow never to be bosses.

When parents renege on authority, parent–child relations are reduced to a power struggle. The father described by Lasch shirks a role of authority at the same time that, ironically, he wears his aggression right on his sleeve, in that he refuses to give his child the punishment he rightfully perceives her not only to want but to need, thus denying her a father who is in the driver's seat. We can hardly call this an act of love. Instead, we can understand it as a passive–aggressive act that masks the father's underlying rage. And, by withholding punishment where it might have helped bind his daughter's adolescent, uncontrollable impulses, the father is engaging in a perverse power struggle in which he refuses to lose to his child. This is precisely what happens in the absence of authority. We are left only with the dynamics of "control or be controlled."

Children are not born civilized. They depend on the environment around them to help bind their impulses and desires so that they can live in the company of others. To accomplish this goal, they at times need to be reined in by the people who care for them. By internalizing a benevolent authority figure who loves but also expresses clear disapproval for transgressions against the norms of acceptable behavior, the child will develop an inner set of controls and self-monitoring. Over time, the child keeps her hand out of the cookie jar not because her hand will be slapped but because she has internalized a sense of right and wrong, of appropriate and inappropriate. But, for a period of time, a parenting figure has to be there to remind her to keep her hands out and to establish consequences when she doesn't.

Without such an evolving structure, life at home is reduced to survival of the fittest. Rather than respectful relationships with generational hierarchies, we have masters and slaves. We all know the story of Cinderella, exploited and abused by her stepmother and stepsisters. But today we have the reverse situation, where the children apparently hold the power and, as one father exclaimed about his two sons, himself, and his wife, "I feel like they're the masters and we're the slaves." In this family, it sometimes gets so bad that the father "loses it" and shrieks uncontrollably at his boys. He temporarily regains control as parent while his boys whimper or cower in fear, and the power positions reverse. But the next day, the tables are turned again as the children demand snacks and dinner in front of the TV, and Father complies so as to be a nice guy, suppressing his resentment and fatigue. Until he explodes again.

Alexis's father was in no better position when he wished that even occasionally his daughter would do something just because he said so. Alexis's mother was left similarly impotent. What ought to be implicit to a child by age four had to be made explicit by Alexis's mother to compensate for the years in which she was trying to be an equal rather than an authority figure to her child: "You're going to do this right now because I said so."

It is inescapable that, when we renege on being an authority to our children, we are periodically reduced to being power mongers to survive our children—reverting to saying, "Do it because I said so." Power, in contrast to authority, is defined more narrowly as the sheer possession of control over another—no need for greater wisdom or respect. Intimidation and fear will suffice.

In such a world, children do things only because someone else makes them, not because they would like to for themselves or for the other person. At other times, the children operationalize their own goal of making someone else do something for them. In the absence of authority, when the only recourse is power, today's parents are left quite crippled in the management of their children. They are well aware of the vagaries and abuses of power. That is why they shied away from being authority figures in the first place. But in moments of pure desperation, they might "lose it" and resort to the position of despot, rather than benign authority, to their children. And then follows great guilt and an even greater avoidance of authority, which becomes misconstrued as dangerous tyranny. So parents find themselves in another impossible pendulum swing, from abdication of authority to power mongering.

Within such swings children are given ample opportunity to turn the tables and seemingly abuse their parents. Child psychiatrist and family therapist Lee Combrinck-Graham reports about a divorced mother of three children, ages eight, seven, and five, who came to see her because of the behavior problems of her seven-year-old boy. Through family therapy sessions, it became clear that the two daughters were acting out, too, calling the mother names, being obstinate, and urinating on the living room rug. The eight-year-old threatened to burn down the house and threw fierce temper tantrums whenever the mother left, even to go to the grocery store. The father claimed to have no problems with the children, and simply threatened to whack them if they got out of line. Mother felt she was a bad mother and that it was all her fault.

The therapist took the tack of asking the mother why she put up with so much abuse from her children. She even suggested that the mother might want to give them up for adoption. The mother was shocked. The children proved the therapist's point by acting out and abusing the mother right in the therapy room. The drama escalated. The therapist reports: "Suddenly Mrs. Putney snapped. She shouted, 'I don't know why I should have to put up with this! Sit down, Peter, or I'll shake you. Shut up, Pamela, and don't *ever* let me hear those filthy words out of your mouth again! How dare you treat me like that! Who do you think you are?' " The drama continued until the children began to cry. Then Mrs. Putney cried, too, and gathered her children to her and talked to them about the need for their cooperation if they were going to make it as a family.[14]

The rapprochement that followed the mother's angry outburst is a nice example of the reparative effects of a parent finally taking over as an authority figure to her children, confronting their behavior in firm words that let them know she means business. If the interaction had held fast at the level of yelling and counterprotests from the children, the dynamic would have remained frozen at the level of power mongering. But the ability of the mother to fuse aggression with love and hold her children close to her as she explained what she needed from them drew this scenario to a healthy close. Now the mother could be a legitimate authority and the children were freed from the relentless power trips with their mother, driven by an unconscious attempt to achieve exactly what was accomplished with the facilitation of an outsider—the establishment of Mrs. Putney as a parental authority figure for the benefit of both herself and her children.

The story of Mrs. Putney, a divorced mother struggling to keep her family of three children afloat, reminds us of another reality that must not be overlooked. *Social* as well as psychological forces intrude on parents' ability to exercise authority with their children. A recent article, "The Battle of Bedtime: Children Win but Late May Not Be Better," documents how children's bedtimes are getting later in the United States. Some of this is accounted for by working families, as later evening is the only time they get to see their children. But another variable comes into play: "Some parents are unable or unwilling to exert the kind of authority over their children that earlier generations did."[15] Looking not to internal dynamics, but to external stresses, the article suggests that parents who work may be less able to tolerate the crying or protests if they attempt to enforce an earlier bedtime with their children.

The hour of bedtime is really not the major issue. But the new phenomenon of later bedtimes alerts us to the fact that today's parents may lack the resources or the "reserve tank" that it takes to be an authority in face of children's unhappiness or opposition. When we are worn out, we ourselves may be more irritable. We may also be less resilient in the face of others' irritability or anger toward us and will therefore do anything humanly possible to avoid being the recipient of such feelings. We dodge being an authority not only because of our ambivalence about aggression, our commitment to conflict-free democratic parenthood, and our fear of losing our children if we cross them. We are also too pooped.

We need to find ways to take command, make judgments, and set examples, rather than succumb to the battle fatigue incurred by the difficult task of balancing work and parenting, which leads us to do anything to avoid another war encounter. We do have other options. It involves taking the long view rather than the short view. It may be totally exhausting to lock horns over a household chore or TV program tonight, but if you put in the extra effort now, the pay-off will be smoother evenings down the line. It's a faulty equation to think that retreat preserves energy. It simply exhausts you in another way, as you brace yourself to return home each day to a child who seems to want everything and stop at nothing. Mustering up your resources and calling on your reserve tank of energy will have just rewards—a child who is contained and respectful and a pleasure to come home to after an exhausting day rather than a child who is impulsive or needy. And there will be the added prize of a family cadence that emanates harmony rather than chaos or friction.

If we can overcome our own fear of aggression, relinquish our allegiance to our own fraying youth status, and find a way to call on a "reserve tank" of parenting energy, we will do much to enhance our ability to become legitimate authority figures to our children. We must also get a grip on our fear for the future and our lack of confidence in our child-rearing strategies and behaviors, for that only exacerbates the problem—we relinquish authority because we do not feel very wise and do not know into what world we are leading our children.

Our own children's protestations of "It's not fair" or "You're not my boss" do not often enough meet with an understanding but firm reply from us: "Yes, it's not always fair and yes, I am your boss." Until we can do that, we will find ourselves in deep trouble when it comes to setting specific limits with our children, a problem to which I would now like to turn.

DISPELLING THE DANGERS OF DISCIPLINE

Today's parents are maligned for not taking the energy or the time to provide guidance for their children and to bring them back in line when they begin to go astray. Never home and too preoccupied to attend to their children when they are, the new parental mode is perceived as opulent neglect. Without also taking into account the larger societal ills that might lead children astray, this becomes an unfair aspersion on parents' characters. Society and parents' psychology feed off each other, and neither is solely to blame for children's going astray. But we cannot deny that contemporary parents are indeed not on firm footing when it comes to the issue of "discipline."

In good enough parenting, discipline is not divorced from but is part of parental love. It is governed by the desire to have our children grow up to be responsible people who both "contribute in" and find success in their lives. It involves reminding our children every day how to behave to become that kind of person.[16] It goes beyond establishing strong emotional bonds, being a good role model, and educating our children about our beliefs. As part of discipline, we make note of our children's successes and place negative sanctions on behaviors that would lead them in an opposite direction. Although overall societal values certainly pertain, a very strong subjective factor also governs as each family determines what kind of person they want their child to become and what strategies they employ to move their child in that direction.

I have already documented how much we want our children to make it in this world and how anxious we have become that they will not meet with success. So the motivation that propels parental discipline is strong within us. Where we need help is in the everyday practices—the limit setting, the enforcement of consequences, and the "management" of the child. We keep collapsing under the demands of being disciplinarians to our children. When it comes right down to it, we are wimps. Whether our children are age two or eighteen, we can get the help we need through asking ourselves, "What is my child trying to tell me here?" and "What should I do to give my child what he or she needs?"

Story One: The Boy with the Noose around His Neck

Craig and Marcia came to consult me because their six-year-old had threatened to kill himself. They were extremely worried that their child might be seriously disturbed, perhaps suicidal. What had six-year-old Jason done? After an altercation with his mother over whether he could watch more TV (Mom had said "No"), Jason took a rope, tied it around his neck, and said, "I'm going to hang myself." I asked the mother what she had done when he appeared with the hangman's noose. She explained that she had turned to Jason and said, "Oh, I would be really sad if you did that." Losing grip of my professional neutrality, I responded in astonishment, "You mean, you didn't first take the rope off his neck?"

If Marcia had thought this was all a joke, a bluff on Jason's part, she would not have been in my office consulting about Jason's possible suicidality. Because she did think it was serious, her message to Jason in setting no limit on his hangman behavior becomes, "It's your life, kid." In an effort to respect his autonomy and not impose her own will, Mom totally forgot to first protect him by setting a limit in response to his rebellion of her prior TV limit—no ropes around necks.

Story Two: Dickface

David, who was nine, had taken to yelling "dickface" at his parents, Joanna and Lester, on a daily basis. The novelty was wearing thin. They were at their wits' end. I asked them what they did when he began his town cry. They explained how they communicated to him that "dickface" was not a nice thing to call someone. Effect: Zero. I suggested that they now tell David, with unflinching authority, to knock it off. End of discussion.

Joanna and Lester, on their next visit to me, expressed their great appreciation. "Dickface" had stopped. Joanna turned to me, with tears in her eyes, and told me, "Thank you so much. You gave us back our power." In my head, I heard my own mother say, "And for this you get paid?"

Story Three: You Can Always Leave Home

Robert and Emily came to see me very distraught about their son, who had just graduated high school. In three weeks, Brian was leaving for his first year at college. By his parents' description, he had become "an irresponsible jerk," impossible to live with. They described it as a Dr. Jekyll and Mr. Hyde transformation. This fine, upstanding high school student was now not coming home at night, taking the family car without permission, and failing to do his assigned chores at home. To make matters worse, everywhere the family went together, he would announce loudly and clearly to all who would listen that he could not wait to get out of his parents' miserable clutches and on to his own freedom. In the process, he said some very hurtful things about his family.

I first helped Robert and Emily recognize that their young Mr. Hyde was just expressing his anxiety about leaving home and entering college (I was able to confirm this because I had previously worked with Brian). On the other hand, that still did not excuse his inconsiderate and irresponsible behavior. I counseled the parents to set down a limit. If he wants his freedom so much, he can have it three weeks early by moving out now. But if he wants to be part of the family for the next three weeks, he'll have to abide by the household rules and stop his public displays of parent bashing.

Emily became tearful. Her head said this was good advice but her heart reeled from the implications of so precipitously snipping the apron strings. Robert, on the other hand, himself a corporate business executive in charge of hundreds of employees, remained composed and calm. Nodding his head, he mused, "I get it, it's like firing someone." Not quite, but it is about asserting yourself and not letting your children mow you down.

In each of the three stories I might very well sound like the hard cop, the enforcer, telling parents to get tough with their children. It is not how I like to think of myself, either as a professional or as a mother. I reassure myself by recalling all the times I counsel parents to be less harsh and punitive toward their children, to soften up in their interactions. I think of the painful moments when I work with a parent who can hate more easily than love and harm more readily than help. But these are not the parents we are talking about here. Our focus is on the underaggressive ones. With these mothers and fathers, I do find that I have to lend them some measure of personal aggressiveness to get them on track to manage their children, whether four years old or eighteen. It is not often a question of giving them *back* their power, but helping them discover something entirely new, that is, abilities in limit setting that they have never possessed before.

• • •

DANGERS FOR THE UNDERDISCIPLINED CHILD

Parents shirk from disciplining their children and often can take charge only with the gentle prodding of an outsider. Over the years, mental health professionals working with parents of children with psychological difficulties have noted that while the child is perceived as being in a state of illness, parents shy away from imposing limits on their child. In a footnote to a case analysis presented by Winnicott, he commented: "[Parents are having] difficulty in [the] management of [an] ill child who is recovering: the question, when to be firm and act on the basis of the child's being normal? i.e., [helping the child's] recovery . . . toward being a spontaneous child in the family."[17] Another practitioner, Hugh Clegg, remarks in his book *The Reparative Motif* that parents of difficult or nervous children who are presented for treatment are often hesitant to exert any kind of influence at all on their child lest they cause irreparable damage in their ministrations.[18]

Certainly, if children are in a state of acute depression or anxiety, it would be insensitive to demand they be as accountable to parental expectations as when they are well. But observation of parents with their psychologically ill children poses a critical question about all parents today. Could it be that modern parents are remiss in disciplining their children not just because they are aversive to roles of authority and expressions of aggression but also because they see their child in a perpetual state of "illness" for which they are trying to compensate? Recall that parents err toward doing too much for their children to correct for feeling that they have not done enough. We also equate any type of suffering with illness and worry that inflicting our authority will create suffering, which will exacerbate the illness already incurred by not having done enough for our children. In an unsafe world in which a parent does not feel sanguine about a child's future and simultaneously worries about the child's present state of well-being, it makes sense that we would inadvertently slip into an attitude toward our children, albeit unconscious, that they are not well and therefore need to be treated with kid gloves. In the wounding of parental narcissism, we believe that our children are wounded as well.

If this is the case, we need to correct it, for, as Winnicott points out, it prevents our children from living spontaneously within the family and inhibits their full development as normal, healthy beings. Further, if we have a child who is indeed expressing psychological difficulties, it may well be that the illness is exacerbated or even caused by the parents' inability to set limits and enforce discipline. In that case, the remedy is the very enactment of disciplinary strategies that were missing before. The story of "dickface" is a case in point. His parents' laxness made him "sick," their firmness got him "better." The equation is as follows: The underaggressive adult becomes an undercontrolling parent who creates an underdeveloped child. This is not good. (Some parents feel so helpless to discipline their children that they send their adolescents off to mental hospitals because that is their last resort of containment when they can no longer control their child. Their hope is that the hospital will be able to do what they could not.) Better is the parent with a healthy integration of personal aggression and love for the child. This is the parent who knows how to place age-appropriate expectations and controls on the child's behavior to facilitate a child's healthy sense of self and good development of internal controls so she or he can make a go of it in the world.

But parents will only be able to do this when they can get over their own fears of breaking their child's will with a hand they feel is too firm. As long as they are indulgent and set few limits on their child, they are both abnegating their own needs and presenting to the child an adult who is self-effacing and even self-obliterating. Although they may believe they are being respectful of their child by not imposing their own will on a weaker being, the false sense of victory for the child is ominous. Children discover that whatever they want, they can get; whatever they do, there appear to be no consequences. In their inner fantasies they imagine they have destroyed the parent, which of course leaves no one driving the bus. The children will then push harder to impose their will, in a desperate attempt to resurrect the parent and find someone in command there.

Jessica Benjamin, in *The Bonds of Love,* describes the effects of the permissive parent who begs off on any kind of discipline:

> The parent has ceased to function as an other who sets a boundary on the child's will, and the child experiences this as abandonment; the parent co-opts all the child's intentions by agreement, pushing him

back into an illusory oneness where he has no agency of his own. The child will rebel against this oneness by insisting on having his way even more absolutely. The child who feels that others are extensions of himself must constantly fear the emptiness and loss of connection that result from his fearful power. Only he exists; the other is effaced, has nothing real to give him. The painful result of success in the battle for omnipotence is that to win is to win nothing: the result is negation, emptiness, isolation.[19]

This is not what we intended for our children. We want them to be happy and secure, not empty and isolated. But our unwillingness to give our children a hard time once in a while and our tremendous aversion to invoking our will can backfire on us. In an effort to remedy a harsh situation in which a child's will is broken and in which the child responds only by submission, we risk creating a child incapable of mutual respect because the child has the reverse experience of breaking the parents' will. It is not healthy for children to experience their mothers and fathers as hesitant, guilt ridden, and submissive toward them. With no limits to their grandiosity, the children will experience themselves as flying off into space. No walls will be there to contain them and no sure boundaries exist to bump up against. We will do our children a big favor if we can feel freer to set limits: We will curb our children's grandiosity, facilitate the development of internal controls, and give them confidence in a world that has a healthy balance between love and personal aggressiveness.

The untoward results for the child when this does not happen can be quite serious. A grade school teacher of twenty years describes it well: "Sometimes it seems like there is no bottom line anymore. I have some kids who yell 'child abuse' if you discipline them. They know taglines, but they don't know the lines they cannot and should not cross."[20] A family psychologist with whom I work reported the case of a child who was failing miserably at school for just these reasons. She could not tolerate the rules and regulations at her school, which by present standards were actually quite liberal and permissive. She seemed to be having no such problems at home, and the psychologist wondered with the girl why this might be so. The child readily responded, "It's easy. At school the rules are unbendable, you just have to follow them. At home it's different, because you get to bargain." And bargaining is exactly what this child was allowed to do with her parents, ad infinitum, until there was nothing left with a firm boundary around it. Her constant power plays were not received well in school in a class of nineteen other children, nor did they ultimately leave her feeling happy or satisfied. Rather than tear down the rules at school, the psychologist helped the family tighten them at home, and the child indeed did better. Her mother and father took on a critical responsibility of being a parent—knowing that you *are* the boss and that you have to be ready to take the heat.[21]

When parents are remiss in setting limits, children are given a false sense of efficacy. They may feel inflated in their bargaining powers, but lack any sense of accountability or sensitivity to others. They are impeded in their abilities to employ internal brakes on their urges and impulses, and they are given an artificial sense of adulthood and freedom, which too often deteriorates into tyranny rather than love and manipulation rather than give and take. They themselves can grow tired of all the permissive parenting, and can finally explode with, "Just stop me." It would do well, then, if the underaggressive parents today could tighten their seat belts, fortify themselves for an occasional bumpy ride, and recognize that love with no firm parental wall to which children can respond leaves a child anxious, self-centered, and aggressive, rather than healthy, wealthy, and wise.

CHAPTER NINE

· · · · · ·

The Kinderdult

*For all the din and flutter from new electronic
stimuli, and for all the leering ads that exploit
youthful sexuality, children experience life
differently than we do. Adults may try to impose
themselves on children, but the children still live in
their own world, with its own set of values . . .
they deserve to be listened to on their terms, not
ours. For the sake of the children.*
　　　　—For the Sake of the Children, THE NEW
　　　　　YORK TIMES MAGAZINE [Special Issue][1]

Up until now we have looked at the challenges of child rearing from
the viewpoint of the parents, giving only brief attention to the effects
of perilous parenting on the child. Who are the children of these
mothers and fathers who parent too much to compensate for parenting too little? What is their own experience of their childhoods? Who
will they become when they grow up? It is time to look at life from
their perspective.

　We know that over the last decade adults have grown increasingly
concerned that today's children are being robbed of their childhoods.
A mother laments the Lolita look among little girls today: "It's not
really that I want her to be a little girl forever. It's just that it would
be nice if she were a child during her childhood. Instead, she's bathed
in the fantasy of bodies and beauty that marinates our entire culture.
The result is an insidious form of premature sexual awakening that
is stealing our kids' youth."[2] Children strutting their wares, dodging
bullets, home alone, or caught in the fast track are all seen as boys
or girls whose childhoods have been foreshortened, or denied to them

altogether. How ironic that the Peter Pan generation, dedicated to the preservation of youth, should have produced a generation perceived to be deprived of theirs. Or have they been?

In 1993, *The New York Times Magazine* published a cover story, "Little Big People." A photograph on the front cover displays three children posed to make the point—the young male executive, the childish femme fatale, and the little jock with his Gameboy. The byline on the cover reads, "Little Big People / They're precocious, even out of control, and their affluent parents have only themselves to blame." The author of the article, Lucinda Franks, explains it as follows: "Today's crop of under-12's, particularly in the middle- and upper-middle-income families and particularly in urban America, seems to have reinvented—or even bypassed—childhood as we knew it. . . . They are proud, independent, and strong-willed; they are worldly-wise and morally serious. They are a generation that has been raised to challenge and doubt authority, to take little at face value—in short, to enter the world of maturity long before they are mature."[3]

On two counts, this depiction of children today is inaccurate. First of all, it is not the children who have invented a new concept of childhood. They are simply the product of the social world that outlines the parameters of childhood for them. It was certainly not them but the clothing industry that designed miniature versions of femme fatale clothing, and not them, but their parents, who foot the bill for such purchases. Secondly, only one side of the equation is being looked at. Yes, today's children are treated as miniature adults, but they are simultaneously considered little cherubs, far removed from the responsibilities of adulthood or even traditional childhood. And they do have a childhood, it is simply different than the one we had. It is a split experience. While mothers and fathers are sergeants by day, fairy godparents by night, children, too, have their divided existence—independent superstars by day, coddled angels by night.

My children are grown and living on their own, with my youngest now in college. I now have time to reflect, to take the long view on their childhoods in light of all the issues I have been writing about in this book. These two children I raised—did they or do they show signs of the kinderdult, half cherub and half miniature adult? Looking back at each of my children, two images stand out.

Rebecca, age twelve, has been invited out for dinner with her grandparents at an elegant hotel restaurant. She waltzes down from her room, radiantly beautiful, standing proud in her first pair of high-heeled shoes and sophisticated "going out" dress. She is showing the lovely new curves of early adolescence and the fruits of her first experimentation with makeup. In her arms, she clutches a teddy bear.

Jesse, at age sixteen, travels independently from California to Kenya to join a summer community service program. There, in a small village, he lives on his own in a house of brothers and helps build a schoolhouse for the village children. Two years later, he calls us long distance from college to assist him because he cannot figure out how to dial information to get a telephone number. In essence, we remain his directory assistance. How could both be true? While away from us, he developed many skills of independence at an early age. But within the walls of our own home, his father and I were all too eager to take care of things for him to make up for all the time we were away from him and to relieve him of pressures we felt were upon him. In the process, we were quite uneven in teaching him the skills that would prepare him to be a grown-up. So now he is a competent young man and a worldwide traveler and is occasionally like a small child in need of assistance.

All of us hold our breath throughout our sons' and daughters' childhoods, wondering if they will make it out intact. We are a generation of intense worriers. If my experience of my own children emerging from that journey can serve as a soothing voice to all of us, I'd like to share that story. Despite strong evidence of the kinderdult within them, my children have turned out to be fine human beings. They are bright, empathic, enthusiastic about life, and confident. They have clear goals about where they are going, have had many culturally enriching experiences throughout their lives, and want to make a difference in the world. They feel fully respected within the family and have room for their say-so. They show great love and respect for us. All this in the context of two baby boomer parents who were as conflicted and guilt ridden as any of the families addressed in this book.

No doubt, their healthy entrance into early adulthood has not come without its bumps and spills. Are my children the exception rather than the rule? Whereas I certainly like to think of my children as special, in many ways they are also typical. As I watch them and their friends embark on the rest of their lives, I would like to give credit to our generation for having done something right by our children. Our efforts to break down generational barriers, be more emotionally accessible to our children, and recognize their worth as vital beings in the world have borne some good fruit.

Our children are inquisitive, resourceful, self-assured, and competent in the world. Children of this generation who have been given credence about their abilities and a respectful place in society have been able to do wonderful things. For example, four hundred eight- to eighteen-year-olds developed a TV news program, "Children's Express News Magazine." It covered such issues as standards in psychiatric hospitals for adolescents, political campaigns, foreign debt, and abortion rights. The children published a magazine, had a syndicated news column, and put together a book containing a collection of their best articles.[4] Elevating their status has certainly had its rewards.

At the same time, it has had its problems, too. Too many children come into my office collapsing under the strain of trying to be ten-year-old adults. Others come in looking like pieces of a puzzle that don't fit together. I am particularly thinking of a fourteen-year-old girl who was sent by her single mother because she kept breaking all the family rules and seemed hell bent on holding wild parties in her mother's absence. Yet she still liked to climb in bed and sleep with her mother every night. She sat cross-legged on my office floor, wearing a push-up bra and décolleté T-shirt, earnestly playing Catch-a-Fish, a game for "four years and up." Femme fatale and four-year-old wrapped into one.

The kinderdults are not in *grave* danger, but they do face many risks and shoulder heavy psychological burdens, different from the ones many of us had growing up in the 1940s, '50s, and early '60s. They traverse through a childhood riddled with contradictions. A whole market has grown up around their specific needs and wants, but they go to school to discover one more program cut from their education because funds have been taken away from them. Their moms and dads are scurrying around just trying to get through a day, yet they still find themselves under the microscope of their parents' overzealous scrutiny and concern. In the words of my own daughter, some years ago, "You just don't know what it's like to be a kid today." Now, cognizant of the pendulum swings of parenting and our split concept of childhood, perhaps we can begin to learn.

A MEETING WITH A KINDERDULT

At age seven, Gwendolyn's parents brought her to see me because of behavior problems at home and peer difficulties at school. Her mother and father had been divorced since she was quite small. She would get into snits with other children when she did not get her way. She did the same with each of her parents, particularly her mother. I had two strong impressions when I first met Gwendolyn. My overriding first impression, written at the time, is as follows: "Gwendolyn is a sad little girl, feels old beyond her years, very bright, with a large, pensive, and brooding face. Yet, at the same time, she seems so confused about things, as when she tells me with great assurance that each day she will be commuting to school near the Nevada border if her father moves to Utah so that she will be closer to him." Spending a little more time with her, I was very taken with her sense of industry and competence, and I wrote as my second impression, "Gwendolyn is very industrious. She is self-motivated and goal directed. She draws with a sure hand. This is a girl who is 'going places.' She feels very comfortable reaching into a drawer and choosing colored markers on her own. She has an excellent concentration span, low distractibility."

Then I took a look at the picture she had been drawing, a self-portrait. Gwendolyn had created a very odd portrayal of herself. The figure she drew was extremely top heavy: a well-defined and brightly colored head and torso, a weakly penciled-in bottom from the waist down. Gwendolyn feels as strong as her intellect is strong. But the bottom part of her, symbolic of motility, physicality, and spontaneity, feels more depressed, helpless, and infantile. I began to see her drawing as the perfect representation of the kinderdult, half miniature adult, half baby.

Further contact with Gwendolyn confirmed my perception. Her father explains to me that he tells Gwendolyn she shouldn't cry, it's just a form of manipulation. Her mother appears to want Gwendolyn to perform to her fullest potential, and insists that Gwendolyn continue with her piano lessons, even though Gwendolyn wants to quit. At the same time Gwendolyn is often allowed to run the show at home, with few limits set for her. I describe to Gwendolyn's parents my assessment of Gwendolyn as a child who is both being pushed to the limits of her emotional and cognitive capacity and unnecessarily coddled. That is why she switches back and forth between ages two and twenty in the course of any day. The father perceives the mother, the primary parent, as relentlessly wanting Gwendolyn to be perfect. But the mother's perception of her relationship with Gwendolyn is not at all one of pressuring her. Instead, she describes their life this way: "I devote my whole life to giving this child pleasure. She goes to more celebrations than anyone I know." And Gwendolyn's response to all of this is to act like a baby, throw tantrums, and snap at her mother: "I don't have to do anything you say."

But Gwendolyn has a lot to say about her own life (italics added): "When my mom isn't too focused on herself, she's too focused on me! *Sometimes I feel like a princess who is responsible for nothing and sometimes I have to take care of everything.*"

She also has a notion that life would work better if she and her mother could meet as equals. Gwendolyn does not create this idea of equality out of thin air. She and her mother have household rules, such as not interrupting. If either of them transgresses, the other is allowed to give a warning and then a punishment if the warning is not heeded. Gwendolyn complained to me that she had attempted to impose on her mother a punishment of no sweets for several nights because her mother had broken the interrupting rule. But Gwendolyn said her mother whined, "That's not fair. You didn't give me a warning." When I interpret to Gwendolyn what a burden it might be for a little girl to have to play a parent and mete out punishments when she could be doing other things, she responds indignantly, "But that's the only way I can make things equal and stop my mom."

This false notion of equality is what signals Gwendolyn as the quintessential kinderdult in a modern household. It becomes clearer when Gwendolyn describes the big fights she and her mother get into. Gwendolyn demonstrates with her hands: First things start out equal—Mom and Gwendolyn are on the same plane (hands flat right next to each other). Then her mom starts focusing on Gwendolyn and not on herself and things start shifting (hand representing Mom rises way above hand representing Gwendolyn). Then it gets to a crisis point and Gwendolyn "loses it" because her mom is so far above her.

Gwendolyn puzzles me by telling me that the blowups start out with her mom being "too nice." I ask her what she means. Gwendolyn tries to enlighten me. Last time she "blew" because Mom started "fru-fruing" Gwendolyn in Macy's dressing room. That meant that Mom starting making a fuss about the clothes Gwendolyn was trying on and, in Gwendolyn's mind, stopped treating her like an equal and started treating her like a baby. (I should mention that Gwendolyn has the fantasy that this same mother expects Gwendolyn to find Mom a boyfriend and "make everything work out okay.") At some point, right in Macy's dressing room, Gwendolyn exploded, unable to tolerate her mother's "fru-fruing" for another second.

In her rages, Gwendolyn sometimes pinches Mom, and sometimes she inflicts upon her what she calls "toe tapping," a euphemism for kicking her mother. She sees this as justified to stop her mother, although she doesn't like how she feels about herself afterwards. She complains further that her mother does something else to spoil the equality between them when her mother stoops to the level of a small child and makes fun of Gwendolyn like an eight-year-old would (which, ironically, might actually establish equality as that is the exact age Gwendolyn is at this time). In the same session that Gwendolyn rants about her mother's destruction of the equality between them, she reveals her own worries at school—she has no best friend, she wonders if other children like her at all.

Gwendolyn, the kinderdult, transforms herself from a miniature adult who believes adults and children should have parity to a veritable two-year-old who disintegrates into wild tantrums that give her pleasure and relief from the pressures placed on her, and then back again to the miniature adult. The child who independently calls me at age eight to set up her own appointments is the same child who gnashes her teeth at her mother. She is wise beyond her years. She is just a baby. A child in need of clinical attention, perhaps she is not a fair representation of most children today. If her parents had been better able to get a clear and consistent picture of who their daughter was, she may never have appeared in the pages of this book. But I believe her story highlights the tensions of youngsters today, albeit in extreme form, in their vacillation between the two opposite poles of childhood that we have constructed for them—the cherub and the miniature adult.

The modern child: an independent laborer and a prince or princess. With the increase in the number of families in which no parent is home during the day, emphasis is put on developing children's sense of self-reliance. Reports are given of children not yet in their teens shopping and cooking for the family, scheduling their own appointments, and purchasing their own clothes. "Self-nurturance" is a term adopted among child development and child welfare professionals to describe children's new afterschool independence.[5] With no one to nurture them when they should be nurtured, they are pushed to nurture themselves. But the reports repeatedly neglect to mention the fact that these same children may be asked to do absolutely nothing during the "second shift," when parents return home after a harried day. Then they transform from independent laborers to princes and princesses, as Gwendolyn explains to us so eloquently.

These children experience three major areas of conflict in their life, as a result of their position as a kinderdult: They struggle with a sense of their own identity; their desires and wants can become confused or muted; and their sense of internal safety is jeopardized by the contradictory demands and protections in an unsafe world. Let us look at each of these three issues individually in an attempt to understand our children's childhood from their perspective.

FINDING THE ONE TRUE SELF IN A DOUBLE EXPOSURE

Earlier I referred to a double exposure as an alternative way of understanding childhood today: We have superimposed the miniature adult on top of the small cherub, leaving us with a blurred vision of who our children are. From the child's point of view, his or her own sense of identity the answer to "Who am I?", is first engendered in the reflection back from the parents—who they see their child as being. Is their offspring a prototype of a grown-up or just a small child? If the parents are not clear about this, surely the children will not be.

Identity formation starts at birth, when a baby is determined to be male or female, is given a name, and joins the culture of a particular family or living arrangement. Through a child's internalization of experiences with the surrounding world and a growing realization of his or her own inner workings, an evolving sense of a self that is unique from any other self develops. It is a process that cannot be hurried and that progresses throughout life.

Identity development becomes particularly salient in adolescence, in the transition from childhood to adulthood. During that time, the child expects and is expected to develop a firm sense of who she or he is. There is a search for continuity with who one has always been but also a crystallization of where one is going and who one is becoming as an adult in the world. A time of experimentation, differentiation, and clarification, our children can often look like they are either all over the map or from another planet as they work toward finding their permanent footing in the world.

Vanessa, a verbally precocious eight-year-old, charges into her therapy session in a rage. Her mother had asked her to do some household chores. Vanessa had yelled at her mother, "I won't do it unless you meet all my demands"; "How dare my mother boss me around like I'm a servant or something!" Vanessa proclaims. I ask her what happened next, after she put her mandate out to her mother. She says her mother just started getting mad and gave her the "lecture." Then they got into a verbal exchange. Finally, Vanessa tells me, she exploded at her mother, "You can't make me be a certain way. I've already decided on a certain path. I'm going to dress the way I like, think the way I like, and do things the way I like." Here I was sitting with a young girl whose teenage identity proclamation precociously surfaces in a child four to five years short of adolescence.

But the story continues. At a fevered pitch, Vanessa goes on to tell me that her mother calmed down, and tried to explain to Vanessa that pitching in on household tasks is part of living together as a family. Vanessa wasn't going to fall for that piece of propaganda, and screamed back at her mother, "No, that's a mother's job." Certainly, she begged me, I should see her point of view and stop her mother from demanding so much. After all, she's only a little kid.

Two weeks later, Vanessa plopped into the chair at my desk, chewing on a granola bar. Full of beans, she was insisting that, at age eight, she was old enough to be left on her own for the weekend. After all, she had already stayed alone for a few hours with great success. (One can only guess that she had just seen the smash hit *Home Alone*.)

There being never a dull moment with Vanessa, some time later she burst into my office, again in a snit. Everyone at school is teasing her and her teacher isn't doing one little thing to stop it. Instead, her teacher says that she should take care of it herself. That's absurd, doesn't her teacher know she's only a little girl who's being relentlessly pursued by her tormentors (Vanessa's own words). (Her teacher has already informed me that she absolutely is asking Vanessa to take more responsibility for her own life, perceiving Vanessa as being too dependent on adults to do it all for her.) But as far as Vanessa is concerned, her teacher is either crazy or sadistic to leave her alone out there in the jungle.

Vanessa, the girl with precocious language who reads adult books and will cut her own path and stay home alone for the weekend, is also a little girl who has trouble keeping her impulses under control, feels lonely much of the time, and wants more of Mommy than she ever feels she can get. She has also taken to telling tall stories and insisting that she knows more than her teachers. In a rage, she scratched nasty epithets into a newly painted cabinet at home. Vanessa's overblown sense of her own power and self-determination is modulated or, more accurately, juxtaposed by her sense of herself as a lonely little girl in need of two imaginary companions, one very good and one very bad. These illusory friends keep her company and also remind her of the two parts of herself. One of her imaginary companions is very grown-up, mature, helpful, and cooperative. The other is always getting into everything, abides by no rules whatsoever, and makes life miserable for everyone. We could certainly understand this as the archetypal struggle between good and evil with which every child wrestles in the course of growing up. But for Vanessa it also aptly represents the separateness and lack of integration between the two parts of herself—a precocious preadolescent, a tyrannical toddler.

Vanessa is telling us her experience of trying to shape an identity out of her life as a "kinderdult." Her story is emblematic of the identity crisis of children who are hurried to grow up, but allowed to remain babies. By adolescence, she may find herself part of a peer group who is allowed to have unsupervised parties, even though she may know full well that the parties may get out of control and nobody will take responsibility. Josh, a fourteen-year-old boy who has been given such adult freedoms, in no way experiences himself as an adult. His class is reading *Romeo and Juliet,* and Josh describes his reactions: "Back then kids were expected to be adults when they turned 13 or so. The difference now is, kids don't have to."[6] Hardly robbed of childhood, Josh sees it as prolonged well past the time of his ancestral peers. At the same time, he is given many more adult freedoms than his own parents ever had in high school, but is devoid of any responsibilities. How will this affect his identity?

It will be split: young sophisticate, helpless dependent. The formation of this split identity starts early and ends very late. The problem for the kinderdult is not necessarily the development of a "false" identity, compliant on the outside and hollow on the inside, but rather a *dual* identity that becomes nearly impossible to integrate into a holistic concept of a self. A sense of self as competent, mature, and independent coexists with a sense of self as unaccountable, free, and pleasure seeking. Both can be equally real. Parallel to their mothers' and fathers' oscillations in parenting, the children's own identity becomes a pendulum swing.

This definition of self is one that has traditionally been reserved for adolescents in our society. They are known to catapult from age two to twenty and then back again in a matter of minutes. The swings are understood as a behavioral manifestation of teenagers' state of psychological disequilibrium and their newly erupting hormonal surges. The swings are also believed to be temporary, subsiding by late adolescence. However, within today's child-rearing structures, this definition of self is not just limited to teenagers. Minus the hormonal surges of puberty, the definition now extends to children across the full gamut of ages and stages. Rather than a transitory stage, it may well become the normative definition of childhood identity today. The only difference is that instead of the *wild* swings known to adolescence, we see a more muted vacillation that pervades all of childhood.

Identities are typically composed of more than one aspect of self and even of seemingly contradictory aspects of being. This complexity is only a problem when the discrete aspects cannot be integrated with one another as adulthood approaches or when they leave a young person with an uneasy feeling of disequilibrium. As a result of perilous parenting in a pressured world, we are responsible for engendering in our children a feeling of disequilibrium and splintering that is now extended downward from adolescence and upward into young adulthood. It is as if our children are perpetually caught in limbo between infancy and maturity in their sense of self. We have created this identity crisis through our own inconsistent image of childhood, which is reflected back to our children in our intimate relationships with them as we do too much to make up for being there too little.

IF YOU HAD THREE WISHES . . . ?

A thirteen-year-old writes about her life in the 1990s. She reflects positively about aspects of her life in contrast to what they might have been if she had grown up a generation ago: "I have more personal freedom now than I probably would have had 40 years ago. I can read more books and see more movies than I could have then. . . . As a girl, I have much more freedom. I don't have to wear a skirt to school. And I don't have to use a separate door from the boys or do any of those prissy girl things. . . . I have more choices in my personal life, too—whether or not to even have a husband or kids."[7]

As a child of the '90s, she refers to her elevated status and expanded opportunities. With such an increase of personal freedom and choices, we would expect children's awareness of and pleasure in their own wants and desires to expand accordingly, as children are given more opportunity to exercise their own sense of agency in the world.

But a little four-year-old growing up in the 1990s belies this notion of the child with expansive awareness of and pleasure in his or her own wants and desires. The son of very democratic parents who support all that our thirteen-year-old above has lauded about her liberated life, little Daniel bounds into my office screaming at me, "I hate everything in your office. There's nothing I want to play with here. No, you couldn't get me anything I want to play with here because there's nothing I want."

In child clinical practice, it is often standard fare to ask a child during an initial evaluation, "If you had three wishes, what would they be?" Over the past ten years I have noticed a distinctive shift in children's responses. It used to be that a child would struggle to whittle down a myriad of desires to a mere three wishes. Now a common predicament is that the child is hard pressed to come up with as many as three wishes. Some children reply that there isn't anything else left to want. Others simply become stymied and tell me, "I can't think of anything." This is not just a matter of children being so satiated and having so many of their material and emotional wants met that they have nothing left to long for. It is also a sign of a dampening, diminution, or confusion regarding desire.

If children are divided in their sense of who they are, it becomes difficult for them then to know what it is they want. Periodically throughout development, children show signs of disruptive or disgruntled behavior where nothing seems to be right and nothing seems to make it better. Parents know this only too well. During those times, if we ask our children what they want, they cannot tell us, because they do not know. These states often coincide with transitional points between two developmental stages. The children are about to leave one stage and enter another and have not quite found their bearings yet. In the vernacular, we refer to this phenomenon as "growing pains."

These transitional points could also be understood as shifts in identity, a straddling between two senses of self, as when a child moves from being a preschooler to being a school-age child. The kinderdult today may be caught in a constant transitional stage. Children perpetually struggle to find their footing in the developmental progression through childhood and toward adulthood. From early infancy through adolescence, kinderdults are faced with the predicament of straddling cherub-dom and miniature adulthood. Instead of increased freedom and choices stimulating desire, their perpetual state of having growing pains chokes desire, leaving children unable to come up with even three wishes.

They are further stymied in their sense of desire by the bartering for love and the lack of firm boundaries around them. Melissa Ludtke, who interviewed several children in preparation for a special *Time* issue on children, describes her impressions of the time spent with the children: "Something is missing in the lives of many children nowadays. They are looking for someone—parents, teachers, ministers—to set limits and impose discipline. Without walls to bounce against, children seem lost."[8]

It's no fun for children to be their parents' bosses. When we are remiss in providing for our children the structures that help them bind their impulses, their sense of desire either fizzles because it cannot find direction or explodes in a chaotic expression of unbridled energy that goes nowhere in particular.

Sarah is ten. She is allowed to set her own bedtime. She's allowed to do whatever she wants after school. She tells me that she talks back to her parents whenever she feels like it. It's only fair, because they get to talk to her that way. Her big problem is that *nothing* interests her. She's bored all the time, and spends a lot of time lying on her bed staring at the ceiling. She doesn't cry much, she doesn't laugh much, she just coasts.

Dominick is her younger brother. He, too, has a surfeit of freedom and a minimum of responsibilities. But he never sits still long enough even to know what boredom is. A veritable whirling dervish, Dominick only wants to know what exciting thing is going to happen next, and whenever it happens it's never exciting enough. Then he's on to his manic search for the next thing that might satisfy his desires, although he can never quite tell you what that might be. Both Sarah and Dominick are children at risk for becoming part of a generation in which freedom leaves you nothing to lose, and nothing is really to be gained from wanting.

To desire something is either to conjure up the unknown or to contemplate something that is not already there. This requires a sense of imagination. Our children experience their life as a fast-moving train with scant time for free, unbridled exploration of inner thoughts and experiences. Imagination gets thwarted and with it plummets the capacity to have desires—to suspend oneself in a state where things don't actually exist.

A child who cannot imagine cannot fully want. Add to that a child who does not have a clear image of who she or he is. Then factor in a child who is always in limbo between childhood and adulthood in a world with no firm walls but with undue pressure. It now becomes understandable why children today might have difficulty coming up with even three things to want.

COPING AND CODDLED IN A CRAZY WORLD

Robert is eleven. He was telling me with great excitement about his father's escapades in the 1960s, when he hitchhiked cross-country by himself. After asking me several questions about the youth culture of the '60s, he mused for a minute, and then shared with me, "I'd sure like to go back and live in the '60s for the safety, but I'd never give up the '90s for the technology."

It is no secret to children today that their parents worry for their safety. A mother reflects on the situation of her four children in contrast to her own childhood experiences of playing out on the streets until dusk:

> Children, to be safe, now must be transferred hand-to-hand—from responsible adult to responsible adult, from teacher to crossing guard to babysitter, from carpool driver to soccer coach, from pottery instructor to au pair—like the precious little packages they are, delivered by courteous employees, signed for at the front door. And when they're home with us, they're kept at our sides, trotting on invisible leashes, doted upon like gleaming Pekinese dogs.[9]

The children of poverty are not privy to such luxuries, but instead are locked in their houses to keep them safe from the violence on the streets.

Sam constantly frets about his personal safety. A boy in his class has tested HIV positive. For a week, Sam stayed glued to the TV watching reports of the Polly Klaas kidnapping. Polly was just a year older than him. Every day he dashes home from school at record speed, breathlessly double bolting the front door as soon as he crosses the threshold.

It is taken as common parlance that our children live in a state of fear—fear of violence, of AIDS, of environmental disaster, of family dissolution. Jules Feiffer captured it well in his cartoon of a little boy[10]:

First frame: I don't want to go to school.

Second frame: I'm scared when I come home, my parents will have moved.

Third frame: I don't want to go out and play.

Fourth frame: I'm scared when I go back in, no one will answer the door.

Fifth frame: I don't want to go to sleep.

Sixth frame: I'm scared when I wake up, my parents won't be breathing.

Seventh frame: I don't want to be a child.

Eighth frame: It's twenty-four-hour-a-day guard duty.

A student in one of my classes, Theopia Jackson, wrote a comment in her student journal about media articles addressing children and violence: "Why does a child feel like it is his responsibility to protect himself? What happens to his/her feeling secure that the adults will keep them safe?"[11] She accurately identified the stress put on children to keep themselves safe in a world that the adults caring for them are not able to make safe. I wrote back to her, "Is there a shift then in children's sensibilities of what childhood is about—no longer a 'children's garden' where young people are protected by their elders, but a terrain in which children and adults alike must fend for themselves?"

But then I thought further about the seeming contradiction—children are also now more protected than they were a generation or even just ten years ago. Nine-year-old Adrianna is never allowed to play outside alone, even in front of her own house. Fifteen years ago, I allowed my nine-year-old daughter to walk her younger brother to the local supermarket or to the street of shops about five blocks from our home. Today that is out of the question for the young children in that same neighborhood—their parents see it as much too risky.

These same neighborhood children report to me about all the coping they have to do to ensure their own safety. Byron tells me about "dropping and ducking." He demonstrates by diving under my dining room table. He had just completed the training program at his local public school where the children were taught how to drop and duck in the face of gunfire. I don't think there is a child over four who doesn't answer, "Dial 911," when drilled about what to do in case of emergency when there is no adult there to help them. So all the neighborhood children seesaw back and forth between preparatory coping for calamity and preventive protection from any harm. Their experience alerts us to another facet of their split existence—in the face of danger they are either young sophisticates or small dependents.

Heather, a very sophisticated thirteen-year-old patient, tells me, "When I grow up, I'll be able to say I survived the hardest time in American history—crumbling education system, violence, divorce." Heather goes to a public school with some racial tension and periodic eruptions of violence. Her parents have been divorced since she was three. She herself took an overdose of over-the-counter medication after an altercation with some other girls at school.

But Heather is also driven everywhere she needs to go and is carefully shepherded between her mother's and father's houses. She, like so many of her peers, is a highly protected child, yet, as she tells you in her own words, a child who is highly exposed, either through personal experience or unrelenting media broadcasting, to an unsafe world. For children who are not part of the more shielded middle-class cohort, their experience in urban America may even transform their hopes and dreams from, "When I grow up . . . " to "*If* I grow up. . . ."

The children's experience of having to cope with but yet being coddled against an unsafe world takes its toll on them. They vacillate between feeling small and scared and being competent and in control. In the effort to protect our children by shielding them from actual harm, our precautions also transmit to our child a sense of insecurity—if Mom and Dad want me locked in the house after school, it surely must be a dangerous world out there. At the same time, children know they're on their own—Mom and Dad aren't around that much during the day, so the buck stops with me in keeping myself safe.

An estimated ten million children are alone most afternoons or longer stretches every day. In 1993, a phone line set up in Southern California for children who are alone from the hours of 3 to 5 P.M. estimated it took approximately fifteen thousand calls from children that year.[12] Our children are highly competent to dial the phone, but are also scared or insecure enough to call a stranger for help or solace.

If we ask our children if they think they are living in hard times, they will give us a definite yes. If we ask them if they themselves find the going tough, we can also expect a yes in response. *Who's Who among American High School Students* conducted a poll of over two thousand teenagers listed in the directory.[13] It would be logical to assume that these children would qualify as precocious teenagers on the road to success. However, forty-five percent reported they knew a teenager who had attempted suicide or succeeded, thirty percent reported that they themselves had contemplated suicide, and four percent said they had tried to kill themselves. Indeed, the rate of teen suicide, childhood mental illness, and alcohol use among youth is on the rise. A report from the Carnegie Council on Adolescent Development revealed that the rate of suicide among young adolescents increased one-hundred-twenty percent from 1980 to 1992.[14] A study appearing in the *Journal of the American Academy of Child and Adolescent Psychiatry* in 1993 reported data that, over the past half generation, children's problems had worsened, according to both parents and teachers.[15]

Our generation may have many things to be proud of in the children we have raised. But we do have to take notice when they tell us loud and clear about the pain they are in and the lack of safety they feel, not just in their external world, but in their internal world as well, where hopes and dreams are hatched and belief in the future is instilled. We disrupt our children's well-being when we deliver the contradictory message that they are not safe, by taking so many extreme precautions to ensure that they are. Children are no fools. The meaning of this message does not escape them. Asked to cope but then coddled in response to a crazy world, our children are at risk for internalizing the feelings of craziness, fear, or despair. As parents, we can check our own rising levels of alarm and fear and deliver to our children a more low-key message regarding the steps they must take to keep themselves safe. We can ask ourselves whether we are indeed pushing our children too far in asking them to fend for their own in our absence, and then take measures to correct that, where necessary, such as by hiring an after-school in-home child care provider, even for an older child. Simultaneously, we will do well to curb our tendency to breathlessly grab our children close to our heart when we arrive home as if we are once again relieved to find them alive. Through such means, we can eliminate the contradictory message of coping and coddling and thus protect our children from the ensuing feelings of craziness, fear, and despair. Through such means we will also be responding to our children's more general plea to us to stop our "crazy" pushing/pampering in *all* areas of life as their best protection against anxiety and despair.

WORK AND THE ADOLESCENT KINDERDULT

Teenagers today like to work. As 1990 rolled around, a third of people aged fourteen to nineteen were in the work force. And most of them resemble a boy of my acquaintance named Jared. Every day after school he dashes off to his job at the local video store. He works until 8:00 and then rushes home to do his homework. He gets paid every other Friday. The following Saturday he goes on a shopping spree—he buys the latest CD, picks up a ticket for next week's rock concert, buys a present for his girlfriend. In a few years, he'll be going to college. His mother has increased her work hours and his father has cut down on his business expenses in anticipation of the six-digit-cost of Jared's upcoming college education, but Jared contributes none of his earnings toward this expense.

Jared's story is emblematic of the 1990s teenage wage earner. Contrast it to the story of my father two generations ago. He grew up during the Depression. When he was a teenager, he went to work to help support the family. All his earnings went into the family pot. An outstanding student, he still could not afford to go to college. When he became a father, he wanted his three children to get the opportunity he never had to go to college. We were expected to work during the summers, and our earnings were to be saved to cover our personal expenses during our college years.

His own grandchildren, however, are no longer imbued with the "work and save" ethic. To revisit the issue of children today not being expected to "contribute in," we find that instead they now live by the "work and spend" ethic. The income earned by teen employees overwhelmingly goes to the purchase of personal items—fifty pair of shoes for one teenager, a car or high tech stereo system for another. Embedded in this "work and spend" ethic is the very essence of the kinderdult.

Teens today earn the power of the purse by going out and getting a job. With the growth of the service sector, jobs flipping hamburgers and running cash registers are increasingly available to them. Their paycheck rarely sees the bank for very long, as the new wage earners engage in ongoing consumer binges. Through their earnings they purchase the trappings of modern adolescence.

While the teens appear to be having a good time with all their earnings burning a hole in their pocket, the adults around them worry. Better to let the children work at honest jobs than push them into illegal money-making ventures, but now we have children with a great deal of economic freedom, less time for their studies, and even less time with their parents as *they* now run off to their jobs. There is growing social concern that these children are being prematurely catapulted out of adolescence. As with the hurried child, the problem with the working teens is that they are growing "too old, too fast." In an article by that title, *Newsweek* reporters comment: "Pulled in many directions, parents grant their working children striking amounts of autonomy. Working at the local McDonald's, in short, has enabled many teens to buy out of adolescence."[16] The transition from child to student to wage earner and consumer is seen to occur much earlier today than in past generations. The result, according to a recent investigator of high school employment in New England, is "a truncated youth, difficult to measure statistically, but evident anecdotally, in a dozen different ways."[17]

We circle back to the perception of foreshortened childhood for our sons and daughters. In certain respects, this is true. Teenagers who work are creating their own youthful version of the harried adult. Jared, my acquaintance who works at the video store, always seems to be in a state of exhaustion. He is hard pressed to balance school, work, and a social life with only twenty-four hours in a day, just as his own mother and father struggle desperately to find time for work, family, and a personal life.

But it is hardly an initiation into adulthood when teen earners are responsible to no one but themselves and spend everything they make on nonessentials. The privileges of youth are merely extended when children are given full rein to be totally self-indulgent with their earnings, purchasing for themselves an opulent adolescence and planning for nothing as far as their future goes. On the one hand, they learn responsibility and the hard knocks of the real world as they hold jobs, lose them, or are turned down for them. But on the other hand, they remain the center of the universe, "your majesty, the baby," as they continue to be financially supported by their families and are free to spend their earnings as they like.

I sometimes wonder why more of the teens don't ask themselves why their parents aren't demanding a more responsible accounting of their earnings, either asking them to save for college or invest at least some of it for the future. Surely it must seem odd to them just at the time when they watch their parents tighten their own belts to prepare for the huge college bill looming ahead. But the legacy of bartering for love, the child-centeredness in the family, and the aversion of today's parents to be authority figures leaves the children with a sense of entitlement and endowment. By the time they are teens, they are well accustomed to being the children who are parented by guilt; they've grown used to having no demands placed on them, in compensation for all the demands that are placed on them. So when I ask Jared if he ever thinks about putting some of the money away for college, he says, "Oh, no, my parents are taking care of that. They've always told me that's the least they could do for me." Both parents and children seem to be in agreement that, if the children have been asked to be such competent copers and be on their own throughout their childhood days, the least the children should reap for their years of precocious and long-standing autonomy is the reward of keeping all their independent earnings for themselves.

In a consumer culture, the teenagers are really not that different from the young adults ahead of them, who operate in the spirit of

"If you have it, spend it," or "Celebrate today, because tomorrow may never come." But at the same time, they are the epitome of the kinderdult in their "work and spend" ethic, as they take on adult responsibilities for long hours and then go wild in the candy store with the only limit being the last penny of their pay check.

GENERATION WHO?

Over the first half of the 1990s, we witnessed a raging debate about what to call the young adults who had just entered their twenties. The media picked up the label "Generation X," which has been fiercely protested as a misnomer by the twenty-year-olds themselves. The most recent initiates into adulthood rankle at the suggestion that they are from nowhere and have nowhere to go. They also resent the attributes attached to this label: "High expectation, low-sweat generation"; "filled with self-importance that sometimes borders on cockiness"[18]; anxious, competitive, valueless, money grubbing, conservative, uncreative, back to basics. Whatever we call them, and however we malign them, these young men and women are in fact the first generation of grown kinderdults. How consistent that an unclear image of childhood concludes with an unclear image of young adulthood, leaving us with the dilemma of what to call them. We could not figure out how to see them as children; now we do not know what to call them as adults.

It is ironic that the "Peter Pan" generation should now express concern that the newest generation of adults is stuck in adolescence. How soon we forget, as we now worry about the latest crop of twentysomething adults who don't seem to want to grow up, who balk at the traditional rites of passage—entering careers, getting married, starting families. Why couldn't they be just like us, who didn't want to grow up but *still* went through all the rituals of job, marriage, and family?

At twenty-two, my daughter informed me that none of her friends were working in their area of study after receiving a BA. Their college degree earned them entry into waitressing, bartending, or low-paid child care positions. In 1994, MTV conducted a poll of sixteen- to twenty-nine-year-olds to discover that one in three young people with jobs think they are overeducated for their present job, less than half believe they are on a solid career path, and half doubt they will achieve their career goals.[19] Many still live in their parents' home because they do not have enough income to live on their own.

These are the same children who were escorted to fancy preschools requiring entrance exams. They are the same children who had affluent and material comforts that their own parents, albeit from middle-class background themselves, could never have dreamed of in their own childhoods. But now they are the young adults who are bumping up against a generational glass ceiling. They strongly believe that they may never have it as good as their parents or as good as they had it as young children. My son tells me that he doesn't believe he will ever have a house as nice as ours. My daughter tells me that many of her working friends in their twenties would be living below the poverty line if it weren't for their parents' help.

Imagine being a young adult opening up the newspaper to read that 1.4 million people graduating from college and graduate school in 1991 were facing a recession job market in which the United States lost two million jobs. In fact, that year college graduates entered the worst job market since World War II. Taking a job they are over-qualified for or working in an unpaid internship is not what they had hoped for nor what they had been primed for in their position as "your majesty, the baby" or "my toddler, the doctor."

These grown children would agree with their parents that the parents indeed have something to worry about concerning their children's future. Their children have the highest levels of education in U.S. history, yet there does not seem to be a place for all of them in the stars. The post-World War II economic boom into which their parents were born is a far cry from the present status of the United States as a declining world power. The wounding of mothers' and fathers' parental narcissism during this decline is reflected in their own children's diminished hopes and dreams. A Roper poll of eighteen- to twenty-nine-year-olds in 1994 found that only twenty-one percent rated their future "very good."[20] Four years earlier, a similar poll found that sixty-five percent of eighteen- to twenty-nine-year-olds felt it would be harder to live comfortably than for previous generations, fifty-two percent thought they would have less leisure time than their predecessors, and fifty-three percent reported worrying about the future.[21]

The newly grown kinderdults are aware of the same thing their parents are—that the adult world they are entering does not look so good. The senior class speaker at my daughter's college graduation spoke eloquently to the parents about his generation: "I don't have answers. . . . Think back to your own graduation and tack on AIDS, a staggering debt, the information super toll road. . . . I think it would be fair to say it's never been so confusing."[22] In short, this generation's own hopes and dreams have been pierced by their perceptions of the limitations of the society in which they are striving to thrive.

Like every generation before them, these young men and women will probably want to do things differently than their own parents did. The conditions of their lives are far different than those of their parents, and in modern society the existential struggle to differentiate oneself from one's elders creates an inevitable dialectic between continuity and change from one generation to another. A twenty-four-year-old graduate student speaks for his generation when he says, "When I raise my children, my approach will be my grandparents', much more serious and conservative. I would never give my children the freedoms I had."[23]

He does not want to be a Peter Pan parent. He does not want to get trapped in bartering for love with no stop signs and no limits. More serious and conservative usually equates with more authoritative. In his dreams of parenthood, he reveals what he wished he had more of himself, a more structured, serious, and restricted upbringing. Perhaps, he is going to be more like his grandparents, he and his parenting partner will have to find more time to spend with their children. Perhaps, in doing so, his generation can remedy the split between the miniature adult and the cherub and replace the kinderdult with a more integrated concept of a child, with a unified rather than a divided identity. Then he and his peers may be able to correct the mistakes of their well-meaning mothers and fathers, who aspired to be perfect parents to perfect children in an imperfect world.

CHAPTER TEN

· · · · · ·

Unspoiling Childhood

*Many parents—especially mothers—live like trapeze
artists: always striving to maintain a balance
between opposing obligations, always anticipating
the trivial slip—chicken pox, an evening
conference—that will spell disaster. Most stressful
of all, perhaps, is the perpetual feeling of
inadequacy that comes from never having quite
enough time or single-mindedness to give to work
or to home.*

—PENELOPE LEACH[1]

As I write these final words of *Spoiling Childhood,* I think how ironic
it is that this book should come to a close just as I, too, come to the
close of my years as an active parent. With one child a college
graduate living on her own and the other away at college, I am now
in the "empty nest" stage of life. But the term just does not fit. Better
put, I face an open terrain. I was one of those mothers who balanced
career and family for twenty-two years, with all the accompanying
stresses. There were headaches and horrors, but I loved my time with
my children. Yet I could not even begin to realize how intense it was
until their years at home ended. It was like not knowing how loud
the music was until someone turned down the volume. In the month
after my youngest took off for college, it dawned on me that I had
returned from moonlighting to having just one job. Rather than being
left with emptiness and a sense of loss as to what to do with my
days, for the first time I felt I had a schedule that was humanly
possible to do in the hours I had to do it.

I have a tremendously strong feeling of "Whew, we made it." I lament it went so fast. I lament the time we did not have. I lament the bickering my husband and I got into over doing our fair share of housework and child care. We were fortunate to have jobs that were flexible enough that we could make time for Rebecca and Jesse during the day. It just often meant working long hours into the night. I feel grateful for what we had, but wish for one thing: that our life as parents could have been more laconic or sane.

My life as a parent was always a juggling act in a seemingly no-win situation, for when you juggle, you are likely to drop at least one thing. I am recalling an incident in Jesse's last year at home. I had set the afternoon aside to work on *Spoiling Childhood*. Jesse came home from school early, as he often did on Wednesdays. He was very agitated over an argument he had had with a friend. He clearly wanted to talk. The minutes ticked by as he sat in my study spilling his heart out. I began to feel fidgety, aware of the work beckoning me at my desk. It was not work that absolutely had to get done that day, but writing I had wanted to get started on. In a fleeting moment of self-reflection, I looked at myself and laughed. It was the ultimate irony. There I was, writing a book about the harried parent perpetually juggling work and family and never feeling he or she devotes enough to either. I was also the person Penelope Leach describes in one of her lectures to American educators and parents: "You either stay home with your children and lose and lose, or you go back to work full-time and lose and lose."[2] So there I sat playing out the conflict, listening to my own son as I simultaneously tried to finish my book, which analyzes and proposes remedies for this very plight of the American parent.

As soon as I saw myself in action I could let go of the chain that was swinging me. Who lost? Hopefully no one. Jesse got my full attention. I eagerly immersed myself in his conversation. It seemed we both felt good. He wanted to talk and I wanted to be there, unencumbered. I realized I had plenty of time left to complete this book, but only a few precious months left before Jesse, then seventeen, would no longer be bursting through the door every Wednesday at 3:00.

But I came to this only after minutes of tension and inner conflict. If Jesse had been twelve rather than seventeen, perhaps I would have only seen endless months of distraction ahead of me and have been less willing to give him my writing time. If I did not have the good fortune of a flexible work life that allowed time at home to write, I would not have even had the luxury of taking time from work to give to Jesse. Instead, I might have been away at an office working long hours, worrying all the while that Jesse would have no one with whom to share his teenage travails when he came home to an empty house at 3 P.M. I know, because on other days I *was* working at the office and felt exactly that. We parents are, indeed, too harried.

By following mothers and fathers in the daily ups and downs of parenting throughout the chapters of this book, we now have a clearer profile of parents today. We are having a challenging and confusing time trying to raise the children who are our charge. We expect to parent perfectly but have less time than ever to do it and few external supports to help us. We proceed with no consistent guidelines for healthy child rearing. We rear our sons and daughters in the flux of a redefinition of both parenthood and adulthood. We are faced with a double exposure image of our child—the kinderdult. Accused of being narcissistic, our real problem is that we have been denied the opportunity for the normative narcissism that was to be our parental right in having a child. We find ourselves constantly swinging between pampering and pushing, doing too much to compensate for having done too little. Afraid of losing the love of our children, we have denied ourselves the personal aggressiveness that is a major tool in becoming an effective parent who can shape and direct. Instead, we parent by guilt. Our children, growing up under such circumstances, carry the specific burdens of a divided existence—half infant, half miniature adult. Childhood is at risk for being spoiled. How can we transcend this?

UNHARRYING THE HARRIED PARENT

Just having completed the chapters for this book, I came across a finding from the Families and Work Institute in New York that stopped me short. Researchers asked parents what their children would say if asked how they would change their relationships with their parents. Parents responded, "They want me to spend more time with them." I certainly would have said the same thing. But when they then posed the question directly to the children, the researchers got quite a different response: "We want our parents to come home less stressed."[3]

In a strange way, children are actually validating the experts who have been arguing for the notion of "quality time"—it does not really matter how much time you spend with your child as long as it is good time. But the children's ideas about time spent with their parents are no doubt very different than the experts'. What I hear in their response is this: "Look, you all may be right that our parents aren't around enough, but that's not the worst of it. You should see them when they are. We have a house run by stressed-out, exhausted mothers and fathers, and *that,* not time deprivation, is the worst of our problems. Please, please, unwind these parents of ours." Even the parents who attempt to give so much to their children to compensate for being around so little may be so harried in the delivery of this "gift" that the child's attitude becomes, "Don't give me a little more lovin', just give me a little less stress."

From the mouths of babes, we hear the wisdom of the times—"Fix our parents by making them less harried." From the harried parent to the hassle-free parent, that is what our children long for. Let us heed their recommendation. If we are to "unspoil" our children's childhood, we must reduce this level of parental stress.

IT TAKES A VILLAGE

Hillary Rodham Clinton, our first lady and child advocate, wrote, "Each of us plays a part in every child's life: It takes a village to raise a child . . . children will thrive only if their families thrive and if the whole society cares enough to provide for them."[4]

My own focus has been to help the families, particularly the parents, thrive and to look at what they are doing as their part in the village. All the while, I never forget that always, in the end, it is the children of whom we speak, for parents are parents only because they have a child.

As part of the village, which in our case is all of American society, our experience as parents is an ongoing dialectical relationship between the social forces surrounding us and our own internal lives. So when we think about transcending harried parenting and increasing the odds of a healthier childhood for our children, we have to look both outside and inside ourselves. Some of the fixing is beyond our immediate control. The social conditions under which we parent are less than adequate and need to be remedied if we are to ensure for our children an unspoiled childhood. This calls for a political movement that makes children a priority and parenting a social concern. But some of the fixing lies within the domain of our own homes and our own psyches. This calls for a value shift that transforms our internal feelings, attitudes, and behaviors about ourselves as parents and our children as our progeny.

Children mandate that we make their parents less stressed, and parents tell us that the only way to accomplish this is to give them more time for their families. The lack of time is the underlying virus that causes the behavioral symptoms of parental stress to which children are so acutely attuned. Children want symptom relief, parents desperately want a long-lasting cure to the underlying disease.

Let us imagine a village that was more sympathetic and supportive to our harried parents of today. It would start with a more time-friendly world for mothers and fathers. Workplaces would have shorter work weeks; parental leave packages; and reorganization of the workplace with flex-time, job sharing, and home-based work. In addition, subsidies and tax breaks would be available to families with children to relieve financial pressures. We can imagine a system that would reverse the present fast moving current that just keeps placing more and more work demands on mothers and fathers alike, robbing them of time for their children. Instead, we would find a work world that abides by the unbending universal of child development—children need a parenting figure who is around enough to raise them—and the basic principle of "good enough" parenting—parents who are going to do more than "subsistence" parenting need to have enough time to parent. This means reducing the number of hours mothers and fathers are away at work and providing far more time for their children than parents have right now.

In our transformed village, parents would not just have more time, they would also experience less *external* pressure to do more and more for their children. This too would help them be less harried. As a society, we would have figured out a way to stop the growing momentum that sends one more letter home or makes yet another demand on a working parent to make time for just one more thing that could as well be done by others, or does not even need to be done at all. As parents, we would have recognized our own part in having created the Superparent who flies in with tattered cape and disheveled psyche. In our village, mothers and fathers would have developed the self-awareness and psychological fortitude to resist such pressures. They would be better able to send a "stop" message to the institutions that might be impinging on them rather than drowning in guilt under the demands.

In our enlightened consciousness about parenting, we as a society would have also awakened to the grave error of requiring parents to pay more and more of the price when their sons or daughters have been less than perfect children, as if it wasn't the fault of all of us. We would have recognized the follies of the recently evolved legal strategy that holds parents responsible and demands that they pay for their children's transgressions. We would no longer find court rulings like a recent one in Illinois in which a mother of a truant daughter, who had already been under court order to attend school, was required to accompany her child to school (all day) for thirty days. This, despite the fact that these "negligent" parents had already changed the girl's school, drove her long distances to her new school each day, obtained counseling for their daughter, and meted out strict consequences for each of her truancies. The village, instead, would attend to remedying the failures in the larger social system that might be leading this girl astray, despite all the parents' good efforts. Parents would no longer be forced to pay for all their children's sins, whether of their making or not.

If such a time should come to pass, parents will become less harried because children will become the collective responsibility of parents and society together, rather than the parents' sole burden. We would see better day care options, not just stopgap measures, such as workplaces that have been "flexible" in allowing parents to bring their children to work if other child care options fall through or are not available. We would acknowledge that workplaces are not set up for children and that, in the postindustrial work world, it is near impossible for mothers and fathers to parent effectively when they are working or to work when they are parenting. And we would know that it is near impossible for working parents to relax when they do not feel confident that their children are being well cared for in their absence. We would assure that all the children had their own stable place for education, growth, and development when away from their parents, with consistent, caring, and competent child care providers and teachers who themselves would be adequately paid for their work.

The village I imagine is not just a pipe dream. The social conditions under which we parent are not immutable—they were different before and they can change again. As parents trying to address those conditions, we are agents of change only as part of a larger social movement that can take action to fix what is broken and create the village we dream of. It will take patience, collective responsibility, and a lot of elbow grease.

In the meantime, important fixing can occur right at home. This is the main thing I have learned from my time with mothers and fathers and my own experience as a parent. And this fixing requires less patience, because it is within our purview to make these changes in our psyches and behaviors right now.

As when they tell us to "chill out," our children remain our best teachers in pushing us to make these changes. Not only do they send us important messages, they are also almost as active in shaping us as we are in shaping them. They are superb in getting us back on track when we have strayed too far from the parenting they need. They become symptomatic and bring their parents to professional consultations, to support groups, to friends, to neighbors, to relatives, and to parents' own self-reflection to fix whatever is going wrong. They tell their parents directly, either through words or action, when things are off balance, as when eleven-year-old Max simply walks out of the room when his parents go overboard in praising him. They confront us with the reality that they are twigs that cannot be bent too far. No matter how we define and categorize childhood, a child will always be a child, albeit in culturally and familially determined forms, but in some fundamental ways as the beings they universally are.

Children are not as fragile as we think. Like children's inflatable punching bags that bounce right back after a playful pop, they right themselves in response to our parenting foibles and rebel when their essence is denied them. Only when they get knocked down too many times in the same way are they at risk. The main lesson we can learn from them is to stop seeing their precious beings as so fragile. A diamond is a precious stone but also one of the strongest natural substances to be found. If, instead of fragile flowers, we can think of our children as diamonds in the rough, we will both honor their resiliency and make great strides in alleviating our parental angst.

My work has taught me that we do great service to both ourselves and our children when we shift from worry about damages to belief in repair. Life is not free from suffering and parenting is not free from foibles. I have never met a parent who doesn't do better when relieved of the expectation of being perfect. It releases us from breast beating and frees us up instead to ask ourselves what choices we have to do something differently when things are not going well. I have come to recognize that the best precept for remedying harried parenting is "If you fall down, get up, brush yourself (and your child) off, and try not to fall down in the same way again." In human relationships, the act of reparation, making good on something that did not initially go well, is far better for character building than providing our children a conflict-free, idyllic, "perfect" childhood. It teaches them that real life comes with mistakes, problem solving, and working things through, rather than with magic wands, fairy god-mothers, and elves helping the shoemaker. And it allows us a little margin for error.

The message from D. W. Winnicott consistently soothed me as a mother: Machines are made to be perfect, people are not.[5] Parent-hood is not about perfection, it's about a general level of care and concern, with much leeway for error and transgression. It's fine for our children to be frustrated with us; it lets them know we're only human (and so are they) and that we and they are separate people with separate needs and wants.

But those soothing words were spoiled when Winnicott and almost all the other psychoanalytic professionals around me were also telling me that we parents have full responsibility for whether things will go well or poorly for our children. I couldn't figure out how we were supposed to parent well with this disquieting double message buzzing in our heads: Whatever you do just by relaxing and being yourself will most likely be fine, but whatever goes wrong is ultimately your fault.

I would like to replace this message with a new one: Parents are not meant to be perfect *and* parents are only partly responsible for both the good and the bad. I believe we can alleviate the pressures from *within* us to keep doing more and more for our children if we embrace the notion that a child's constitution and external forces bigger than the parenting environment also play their part in shaping who our child becomes. Parenting by guilt is doing no one any good. Shifting our internal belief system away from "I must be perfect" and "It's all my fault" to "I'm doing the best I can under imperfect conditions with a little person who is special but not fragile" may provide us with a monumental stepping stone toward eliminating parenting by guilt, reducing our harriedness, and bettering the odds of good parenting.

In the absence of this new message, our relationships with our children will remain riddled with a "just due" attitude toward ourselves. I am reminded of a newly divorced mother who told me her four-year-old daughter was being rude, obstreperous, and impervious to directions or prohibitions, and was kicking, hitting, and spitting at her. This mother doesn't do anything to stop it because she believes she deserves what she is getting for having put her child through such turmoil, not just because of the divorce but because of the intense marital discord that preceded it. Along with parental guilt comes this belief in "just due"—I deserve this for having done X to my child. We see it in bartering for love and in the attitude "use the rod, lose the child." The thought is "My child has every reason to hate me, and I must simply wear my hair shirt and take what comes my way."

If we are to heed our children's cry for less stressed parents, our internal work includes radically shifting our consciousness from a "just due" to a "just do" attitude toward parenting. I began this book by saying that the vast majority of parents want to be good parents. And what I have learned from parents themselves is that, despite all the difficulties of parenting today, most parents indeed achieve that goal. There is no need to feel as guilty as they do and there is no need to bare themselves to meted out punishments, from their children or from anyone else, for not being good enough. They are good enough because they love their children and are committed to them. They are good enough because they hang in there and forge the bonds with their children over time, sometimes under very difficult conditions. They become even better when they listen to their own intuition, and respond internally to "It's crazy what we are doing" with a response that comes more from their "gut" than from guilt, anxiety, or "shoulds."

Moving from "just due" to "just do" parenting is not only about "doing what comes naturally." It requires delving into the deepest recesses of our own psychologies. It is my strong belief that self-knowledge and self-understanding are the keys to change or cure.

For example, we have learned that, as a generation that hoped to straddle childhood and adulthood indefinitely, we sometimes have difficulties differentiating ourselves from our children. Our corrective to this is to ask ourselves, "Who am I doing this for, me or my child?" Although not always an easy question to answer, scales grossly tipped in either direction can be our wake-up call to adjust toward a better balance between baby and me. If the scales consistently seem tipped in the direction of "me," we may need to put our child and his or her needs in better focus. If the scales are *always* tipped in the direction of "baby," with no regard at all for "me," parenting may have become self-effacing and overindulgent and may require some more limit and boundary setting.

"Just do" parenting involves putting a stop to bartering for love and developing more confidence that the love is there and will not go away. This in turn necessitates confronting our own internal turmoil—conflict over feeling we cannot do enough for our children to protect them from harm, ensure a good future, or provide enough time, and thus feeling we must spend our whole lives making up for that. Often this conflict goes on at a deep, unconscious level. To expose it necessitates making the conflict conscious. The turmoil is a combination of the piercing of our expectable parental narcissism, our own overly perfectionist aspirations for both ourselves and our children, our guilt for not giving enough to our children, and our tendencies to be indeed self-involved at times. This conflict is then linked to a specific set of overt behaviors: our hesitancy to discipline and our propensity to indulge our children, coupled with our tendency to ask too little to make up for all we cannot give and then to push too hard as an insurance policy for making it in a rough world. Only when we work through this conflict can we eliminate bartering for love and replace it with old-fashioned unconditional love, which is a key to "just do" parenting.

Another solution to our conundrum of doing too much to make up for doing too little is to shift our consciousness to less is more and more is less. Less indulgence will give us more pleasure in both our parenting and in our children. Less lenience will give us more, not less, love. More time for parenting will give us less stress and less anxiety.

This brings us back full circle to the issue of time. We have to face the reality that our sense of foreshortened time for our children is not only externally imposed by the demands of the work world. We must be honest with ourselves and look at our own choices, asking ourselves if we really need to be doing everything on our schedules. If truth be told, we remain a generation that believes we can have it all, even when we experience that it is no longer coming our way as we would wish. If we can have it all, we want to *do* it all, and this does not mesh well with devoting enough time to our children.

Parents are exhausted. Parenting is exhausting. Sometimes work, as tiring as it might be, seems less exhausting than the demands of our children. So we might find ourselves lingering at work once in a while or taking on an extra work project to avoid the pressures at home. Like any "psychological fix," jumping ship on parenting time only leads to a more intense psychological mess for parents and children alike—children and their needs do not go away, the pressures mount, and parents find themselves even more strung out and guilt ridden. Our lives will ease up if we resist the internal urge to grab the most immediate fix.

More time with the children, not less, is what will help turn parenting from hassle to haven. The village certainly needs to do its part in giving us more unencumbered time for our children. Our part is to stop hurrying so much and to let go of the notion that we can do everything.

• • •

MOVING INTO THE TWENTY-FIRST CENTURY

As we approach the twenty-first century, the prevailing belief is that the guiding principle of parenting has devolved from what is best for the child to what the child can tolerate. Actually, the reality is quite otherwise. Parents are juggling—not what is tolerable, but what is humanly possible to provide.

We speculate that as the year 2000 rolls in, the nuclear family as we had once known it will barely exist. Family units will divide and reassemble with new configurations, new birth technologies will permit families to be made in a myriad of ways, and parenting partnerships will come in all different combinations of race and sexual identity. Anthropological data and simple observation at home have taught us that the family is a surprisingly flexible institution. But what is inflexible is the need for consistent caretakers regularly available to raise the children in these families, whatever their structure. In other words, parenting will never be obsolete. But the challenge that faces us now is how to parent and how to alter parenting to fit the changing times, while abiding by certain unbending universals of healthy child development.

At the opening of the last decade of the twentieth century, great hope prevailed. Some dubbed it "the decade of the parent." The belief was that the public would be demanding services for families and children. The age of narcissism was over. It was predicted that a reinvestment in children was on the horizon.

As we take stock in the second half of that decade, there is really no cause for such optimism. A U.S. Congressional leader promotes a plan to place children of poor, unwed mothers in orphanages. Mothers of those children are to be punished for being young, indigent, and single. Parents are working harder than ever and feel even less sanguine about their children's future. The parental leave bill that was finally passed was a good first step but is truly only a drop in the bucket. In 1995, an article appeared on the front pages of a San Francisco newspaper announcing, "Huge Majority of Day Care Centers Called Mediocre: Chilling Report Comes as Congress Considers Cuts."[6] The President of the United States is making pledges to the middle class not just as a political strategy but because he recognizes that they are clearly in trouble. The only cause for optimism is the swelling recognition that something must give soon if we are to be a nation of healthy children and healthy parents.

To prepare for the twenty-first century, strong steps must be taken to enhance our children's childhood, both within the walls of our homes and within the society at large. The village we envisioned will hopefully become the village of the future, one that will put our children in better focus and replace the double image of the kinder-dult with a single image of a child who progresses from infancy to adulthood with stopping points along the way. My contribution to the effort has been to offer a psychological analysis of the plight of parenting today in the context of the social milieu in which mothers and fathers are raising their children. I believe that many of the inner conflicts of contemporary parenting have remained unconscious and, in bringing them to the light of day, I hope I have been able to offer immediate tools that will instigate change. Like charity, a revolution in parenting can start in the home. In that spirit, I believe insight and the transformation of confusion into clarity can serve as a powerful agent of change. Having a map to guide you bolsters your strength far more than traveling without one through unknown terrain that seems fraught with dangers.

There are no easy formulas for unspoiling childhood, and each family's experience will have its own unique spin. The task is more a matter of thinking through situations in new ways and shifting our sensibilities about good enough parenting and good enough children. I hope that this book can play its hand in fostering such a value shift, one that bends our attitudes and behaviors away from "just due" and toward "just do" parenting. It is ironic that I write a book to harried parents who have no time to parent, let alone read a book. But I envision that the experience of taking the time to read this book and discussing it with others might actually begin a major shift toward restructuring one's own sense as a parent and freeing a path to pose questions to ourselves about why we do what we do with our children and what other choices we have. And for those of us who are not parents ourselves or who address our energies to other parents, I hope our values will shift to encompass a more empathic and integrated understanding of parenting under the difficult conditions mothers and fathers are facing today.

• • •

I would like to end with a final message to parents. The social conditions in which we parent must be improved. We can turn to each other for support and to ourselves for self-awareness. We must transform our values so that we can acknowledge ourselves as active agents who are good enough, rather than feeling like passive pawns who are failures. Only thus can we succeed in unspoiling childhood for our children. With our children, we can stop abdicating the throne and accept our position as an adult. Children do not do well with deposed kings and queens for parents. To be good parents, we definitely must give generously of ourselves, but never give ourselves over to our children. It will help us to know that our parental narcissism has been wounded, but it will help us even more to find the means for healing it by turning away from the lament of what our children might not become to a celebration of who they actually are. In our own psyches we can destroy the image of the kinderdult and stop swinging between pushing and pampering. And most importantly, we need more time. If we can make these changes, both parenthood and childhood will thrive.

Notes

FOREWORD

1. A. L. Gessell and F. L. Ilg (1949), *Child Development,* New York: Harper and Company.

CHAPTER ONE

1. Joan Ryan, "Rules of (Keeping Them Under Your) Thumb," *San Francisco Chronicle,* February 2, 1997, p. 10.
2. Bruno Bettelheim, cited in Jon Stewart, "Bruno Bettelheim," *This World, San Francisco Chronicle,* September 18, 1988, p. 11.
3. Regina Dickerson, "What's the Rush?," *Working Mother,* November 1987, p. 155 and 157.
4. Juliet B. Schor (1991), *The Overworked American,* New York: Basic Books.
5. See Thomas S. Luech, "Baby-Boomers: Realities vs. Dream," *The New York Times,* March 6, 1986, for a discussion of the economic realities of baby boomers in the 1980s.
6. Alice Kahn, The Alice Kahn Column, "Rebel with a Tapered Cause," *San Francisco Chronicle,* April 17, 1988, p. A18.
7. For discussion of this issue, see Neil Postman (1982), *The Disappearance of Childhood,* New York: Delacorte Press. The cause of the demise of childhood, according to Postman, resides in the communication needs of our society. As we are no longer dependent on the written word, the introduction of the spoken message and seen image through television, radio, movies, and videotapes renders a separate category of childhood irrelevant. In contrast to reading, which is rarely fully achieved before the

age of reason (age seven), one does not have to "learn" to watch TV, one does not even necessarily need to have acquired language. Anyone can do it, and young children and adults are simultaneously exposed to the same information through the same medium. If reading and the printing press originally ushered in the advent of a separate status of childhood, with the new demarcation of illiterate and literate categories of people, then the advent of the electronic mass media eliminates that demarcation and with it the need or even desirability of this separate status for children.

8. David Elkind (1981), *The Hurried Child,* Reading, Massachusetts: Addison-Wesley.

9. Diane Curates, "Kindergarten Teachers' AIDS Curriculum," *San Francisco Chronicle,* January 27, 1989.

10. Joan Ryan, op. cit., p. 10.

CHAPTER TWO

1. Sigmund Freud (1914), "On Narcissism: An Introduction," *Standard Edition,* Vol. 14, p. 19.

2. Ibid., p. 19.

3. Lynne H. Williams, Henry S. Berman, and Louisa Rose (1987), *The Too Precious Child,* New York: Atheneum.

4. Jonathan B. Levine and Amy Dunkin, "Toddlers in $90 Suits? You Gotta Be Kidding," *Business Week,* September 21, 1987, p. 52.

5. Statistic reported in James Hirsch, "In TV and Films, as in Life, Babies Are in Fashion Again," *The New York Times,* October 12, 1987.

6. Statistics reported in Martha Smytes, "Older Parents: Good for Kids?," *Time,* October 10, 1988.

7. Ad placed in *San Francisco Examiner,* January 15, 1989.

8. For example, see Andrea Sachs, "When the Lullabye Ends," *Time,* June 4, 1990; Barbara Kantrowitz, "The Long Goodbye," *Newsweek,* October 22, 1990.

9. Miriam Elson (1984), "Parenthood and the Transformation of Narcissism," in Rebecca S. Cohen, Bertram J. Cohler, and Sidney H. Weissman (Eds.), *Parenthood: A Psychodynamic Perspective,* New York: Guilford Press.

10. Hillary Rodham Clinton, "It Takes a Village," *Newsweek,* January 15, 1996, p. 30.

11. See Lynne H. Williams, Henry S. Berman, and Louisa Rose, op. cit.

12. Sigmund Freud, op. cit., p. 90.

13. See Bruno Bettelheim (1987), *A Good Enough Parent,* New York: Vintage, and David Elkind (1981), *The Hurried Child,* Reading, Massachusetts: Addison-Wesley.

• • •

CHAPTER THREE

1. Bruno Bettelheim (1988), *A Good Enough Parent,* New York: Vintage, p. 48.

2. D. W. Winnicott (1965), *The Maturational Processes and the Facilitating Environment,* Madison, Connecticut: International Universities Press.

3. Margaret Mahler, Fred Pine, and Anni Bergman (1975), *The Psychological Birth of the Human Infant,* New York: Basic Books.

4. Heinz Kohut (1977), *The Restoration of the Self,* New York: International Universities Press.

5. Daniel Stern (1985), *The Interpersonal World of the Infant,* New York: Basic Books.

6. Jessica Benjamin (1988), *The Bonds of Love,* New York: Pantheon.

7. Christina Day, "Baby Love," *Working Mother,* November, 1986, p. 190.

8. See D. W. Winnicott (1971), *Playing and Reality,* London: Tavistock, for a discussion of the mirroring concept.

9. Andrew Ward, "Pop Culture: A Father Searches for Himself in His Newborn's Face," *Parenting,* April 1996, p. 7.

10. Lucinda Franks, "Little Big People," *The New York Times Magazine,* October 10, 1993, p. 34.

11. Ibid., p. 31.

12. Lynne H. Williams, Henry S. Berman, and Louisa Rose (1987), *The Too Precious Child,* New York: Atheneum, p. xi.

13. See Sylvia Hewlett (1991), *When the Bough Breaks: The Cost of Neglecting Our Children,* New York: Harper Perennial.

14. See Anne Cassidy, "Why Two Kids Are Enough," *Working Mother,* February 1990.

15. Lucinda Franks, op. cit., p. 34.

16. Ruth Steine, "The Choices Mothers Must Make," *San Francisco Chronicle,* October 29, 1992, pp. D3–D5.

17. Anna Quindlen, "Is 'Quality' Time Really as Good as a Good Time?," *The New York Times,* June 9, 1988.

18. Benjamin Spock (1988), *Dr. Spock on Parenting,* New York: Simon and Schuster, p. 124.

19. Melvin Konner, "Where Should Baby Sleep?," *The New York Times Magazine,* January 8, 1989.

20. Work and Family, "An American Family," *The Wall Street Journal,* June 21, 1993, p. R11.

21. Carol Lawson, "When Day Care Begins with the Night Shift," *The New York Times,* March 14, 1993, p. B1.

22. See Sylvia Hewlett, op. cit., p. 129, for an explanation of the concept of adult self-involvement.

23. Jon Stewart, "Bruno Bettelheim," *This World, San Francisco Chronicle*, September 18, 1988, p. 9.

24. Katy Butler, "Baby Boom's 'Super-Couples' Have Money to Burn," Baby Boom of the 80s [Special report], *San Francisco Chronicle*, October 16, 1984, p. A1.

25. Philippe Aries (1962), *Centuries of Childhood*, New York: Vintage.

26. Deborah Hofman, "For School, Children Want Adult Styles," *The New York Times*, August 28, 1989; Mandy Behbehani, "Power Duds for Children," *San Francisco Examiner*, September 3, 1989; Mary Talbot, "Showing Too Much, Too Soon," *Newsweek*, April 26, 1993.

27. Nancy Chodorow (1978). *The Reproduction of Mothering*, Berkeley, California: University of California Press.

CHAPTER FOUR

1. Regina Dickerson, "What's the Rush," *Working Mother*, November 1987, p. 155.

2. Diane Ehrensaft (1987), *Parenting Together: Men and Women Sharing the Care of Their Children*, New York: The Free Press.

3. "More Time for Parenting Means More Stress over Work," *The Wall Street Journal*, March 13, 1991.

4. Juliet B. Schor (1991), *The Overworked American*, New York: Basic Books. Schor reports that a 1989 poll indicated that almost two-thirds said they would prefer to give up some of their salary, by an average amount of thirteen percent; fewer than one-quarter were unwilling to give up any money at all.

5. Cathy Trost and Carol Hymowitz, "Careers Start Giving in to Family Needs," *The Wall Street Journal*, June 18, 1990.

6. Survey as reported in Lynn Smith and Bob Sepchen, "Workers Carve Time with Kids," *San Francisco Chronicle*, August 13, 1990.

7. Janice Castro, "The Simple Life," *Time*, April 8, 1991.

8. Ibid.

9. Juliet B. Schor, op. cit., p. 164.

CHAPTER FIVE

1. Michael Schwartzman (1990), *The Anxious Parent*, New York: Simon and Schuster, p. 276.

2. Sara Davidson, "Kids in the Fast Lane," *The New York Times Magazine*, October 10, 1988, p. 74.

3. John B. Watson, as quoted in Barbara Ehrenreich (1989), *Fear of Falling,* New York: Pantheon, p. 86. Original source: John B. Watson (1928), *Psychological Care of the Infant and Child* New York: W. W. Norton and Company, pp. 9–10.

4. The exact quote from John B. Watson, ibid., p. 9, is as follows: "Give me a dozen healthy infants, well-formed, and my own special world to bring them up in, and I'll guarantee to take anyone at random, and train him to become any type of specialist I might select—actor, lawyer, artist, merchant, chief, and yes, even beggar and thief, regardless of his talents, penchants, tendencies, abilities, vocations, and race of his ancestors."

5. B. F. Skinner (1953), *Science and Human Behavior,* New York: Macmillan.

6. A. L. Gessell and F. L. Ilg (1949), *Child Development,* New York: Harper and Company. In their own words: "The make up of personality depends upon distinctive and innate factors which are so ancient and deep-seated that they cannot with impunity be transcended, even in a highly sophisticated culture" (p. 37).

7. Deborah Franklin. "What a Child Is Given?" *The New York Times Magazine,* September 3, 1989, p. 36.

8. As reported in Daniel Coleman, "Major Personality Study Finds That Traits Are Mostly Inherited," *The New York Times,* January 1, 1986.

9. See E. James Anthony and Bertram J. Cohler (Eds.) (1987), *The Invulnerable Child,* New York: Guilford Press, for a more complete discussion and compilation of data on resiliency in children.

10. Lawrence Diller, "Not Seen and Not Heard," *Family Therapy Networker,* July/August 1991, p. 20.

11. Anastasia Touflexis, "Struggling for Sanity," *Time,* October 8, 1990, p. 48.

12. Janna Malamud Smith, "Mothers: Tired of Taking the Rap," *The New York Times Magazine,* June 10, 1990, p. 38.

13. Lewis Carroll (1960), *The Annotated Alice,* New York: Bramhall House, p. 113.

14. Torri Minton, "Bay Area Parents Feeling Frustrated," *San Francisco Chronicle,* October 1, 1991, p. A1.

15. Alice Miller (1981), *Prisoners of Childhood,* New York: Basic Books, p. 75.

16. Katy Butler, "Baby Boom's 'Supercouples' Have Money to Burn," Baby Boom of the 80s [Special report], *San Francisco Chronicle,* October 16, 1984, p. A1.

17. Emily Mitchell, "Look Who's Listening Too," *Time,* September 30, 1991, p. 76.

18. Nicole Wise, "Educational TV for the Under-12-Months Set," *San Francisco Chronicle,* May 27, 1991.

19. "What Can a Baby See?," Wimmer-Ferguson Child Products, Copyright 1988.

20. David Perlman, "Education of Babies Shown to Boost IQs," *San Francisco Chronicle*, February 10, 1996, p. 1.

21. Anne C. Roark, "Bringing Up Baby Is a Faddish Affair," *This World, San Francisco Examiner*, October 9, 1988, p. 15, 20.

22. Jane Elder, "The Superbaby Burnout Syndrome," *Education Section, The New York Times*, January 8, 1989, p. 32.

23. Sara Davidson, op. cit., p. 52.

24. Diane Curtis, "Kindergartens Get Picky," *San Francisco Chronicle*, May 18, 1994, p. 1.

25. David Elkind, "Miseducation," *Parents*, October 1987; David Elkind (1987), *Miseducation: Preschoolers at Risk*, New York: Alfred A. Knopf.

26. Sara Davidson, op. cit.

27. Sue Mittenthal, "Kindergarten: Starting Older and Wiser," *The New York Times*, November 20, 1986.

28. Anna Quindlen, "You Helped Put 'Human' in Human Being," *The New York Times*, December 10, 1986, p. 17.

CHAPTER SIX

1. Benjamin Spock (1988), *Dr. Spock on Parenting*, New York: Simon and Schuster, p. 37.

2. As reported in Jerry Adler with Pat Winger, Lynda Wright, Patrick Houston, Howard Manly, Alden Cohen, "Hey, I'm Terrific," *Newsweek*, February 17, 1992, pp. 46–51.

3. J. G. Fitzpatrick (1988), *The Superbaby Syndrome*, New York: Harcourt Brace Jovanovich, p. 74.

4. Personal communication from Kitty Moore, my editor at The Guilford Press.

5. See E. James Anthony (1982), "The Essential Human Child and His Cultural Counterparts: An Epilogue for an International Congress," in E. James Anthony and Colette Chiland (Eds.), *The Child in His Family: Children in Turmoil: Tomorrow's Parents*, New York: John Wiley and Sons, pp. 309–326; for a discussion of the essential child.

6. "Are Children Now Lacking the Time Just to Be Kids?," Wall Street Journal Staff Reporter, *The Wall Street Journal*, January 19, 1988.

7. Piraro, "Bizarro," *San Francisco Chronicle*, August 27, 1995.

8. Donna Cole, "You Could Look It Up—But Don't," *Newsweek*, October 4, 1993, p. 22.

9. This story was reported by E. James Anthony as coming from the work of anthropologist Ruth Benedict. It can be found in E. James Anthony, op. cit.

10. As explained in the book *The Too Precious Child,* "Youngsters today are pressured to get into the right nursery school, the right computer camp, the right college, yet they are rarely required to do anything that would be truly important to the real world" [Lynne H. Williams, Henry S. Berman, and Louisa Rose (1987), *The Too Precious Child,* New York: Atheneum, p. 188].

11. For a fuller discussion of this, see D. W. Winnicott (1963), "Morals and Education," in *The Maturational Processes and the Facilitating Environment,* Madison, Connecticut: International Universities Press.

12. Steven Waldman and Karen Springen, "Too Old, Too Fast?," *Newsweek,* November 16, 1992, pp. 80–88.

13. Ibid., p. 80.

14. See Alice Miller (1981), *Prisoners of Childhood,* New York: Basic Books, for discussion of children who suffer from this.

CHAPTER SEVEN

1. David Elkind (1994), *Ties That Stress,* Cambridge, Massachusetts: Harvard University Press, p. 227.

2. See Margaret S. Mahler, Fred Pine, and Anni Bergman (1975), *The Psychological Birth of the Human Infant,* Part II, New York: Basic Books, for a discussion of the concepts of the fear of loss of the object and fear of loss of the love of the object in early human development.

3. See Margaret S. Mahler, Fred Pine, and Anni Bergman, ibid., for a discussion of this "rapprochement crisis" in the second year of life.

4. "Boy's Bid to 'Divorce' Mom," *San Francisco Chronicle,* September 25, 1992; Anthony DePalma, " '12-Year Old Wins 'Divorce' from Parents," *San Francisco Chronicle,* September 26, 1992; Mitchell Landsberg, " 'Divorce' from Mother not a Likely Trend-Setter," *San Francisco Examiner,* September 27, 1992.

5. For a discussion of this phenomenon of fear of children's rejection, see Bruno Bettelheim (1987), *A Good Enough Parent,* New York: Vintage.

6. Margaret Brownley, "A Tale of Two Mothers," *Working Mother,* September 1987, pp. 111–112.

7. Statement quoted in Jerry Carroll, "What to Do with the Kids?," *San Francisco Chronicle,* November 17, 1993, p. B3.

8. See Glenn Collins, "A Survey of Parents' Views," *The New York Times,* September 26, 1986, p. B1.

9. Daniel Goleman, "What Do Children Fear Most? Their Answers Are Surprising," *The New York Times,* March 17, 1988, p. Y21.

10. Ann Remley, "From Obedience to Independence," *Psychology Today,* October 1988, pp. 56–59.

11. Personal communication from Dr. Eileen Keller, October 1992.

12. Personal communications from Bonnie Rottier, November 22 and December 6, 1993.

CHAPTER EIGHT

1. As cited in Patricia Leigh Brown, "New Magazines for Parents Reshape the Family and Vice versa," *The New York Times,* August 19, 1993, p. B1.

2. Barbara Samalin, as quoted in Jerry Carroll, "What to Do with the Kids," *San Francisco Chronicle,* November 17, 1993.

3. Thomas Gordon (1970), *P.E.T.: Parent Effectiveness Training,* New York: Plume Books.

4. Christopher Lasch (1979), *The Culture of Narcissism,* New York: W. W. Norton and Company, p. 179.

5. Ellen Hopkins, "Abusing the Rights of Parents," *Newsweek,* October 18, 1993, p. 26.

6. For a further discussion of the relationship between love and aggression, see D. W. Winnicott (1950–1955), "Aggression in Relation to Emotional Development," in D. W. Winnicott (1958), *Through Pediatrics to Psycho-analysis,* New York: Basic Books, pp. 204–218.

7. I am borrowing this term "intimate edge" from Darlene Bregman Ehrenberg, which she uses to describe the relationship between therapist and patient in which there is a strong connection but a firm understanding on both persons' parts of the differentiation between the two people in the therapy room together [Darlene Bregman Ehrenberg (1992), *The Intimate Edge,* New York: W. W. Norton and Company].

8. D. W. Winnicott, op. cit., p. 204.

9. Anne Remley, "From Obedience to Independence," *Psychology Today,* October 1988, pp. 56–59.

10. *The American College Dictionary* (1962), New York: Random House, p. 84.

11. Benjamin Spock (1988), *Dr. Spock on Parenting,* New York: Simon and Schuster, p. 134.

12. Christopher Lasch, op. cit.

13. See Anna Freud (1965), *Normality and Pathology in Childhood,* New York: International Universities Press, p. 8, for reference to this

phenomenon in children raised by parents informed by more modern psychoanalytic principles in which parents attempt to reduce the children's fear of them.

14. Lee Combrinck-Graham, "Holding Children Accountable," *Family Therapy Networker,* July/August 1991, p. 51.

15. Trish Hall, "The Battle of Bedtime: Children Win, but Late May Not Be Better," *The New York Times,* March 1, 1990, p. B1.

16. See Benjamin Spock, op. cit., Chapter Six: Discipline, for a further description of discipline as a part of parenting.

17. D. W. Winnicott (1977), *The Piggle,* Madison, Connecticut: International Universities Press, p. 97.

18. Hugh Clegg (1984), *The Reparative Motif,* New York: Jason Aronson.

19. Jessica Benjamin (1988), *The Bonds of Love,* New York: Pantheon, p. 35.

20. Lucinda Franks, "Little Big People," *The New York Times Magazine,* October 10, 1993, p. 32.

21. Personal communication from Dr. Anne C. Bernstein, November 1993.

CHAPTER NINE

1. "What Grown-Ups Don't Understand about What It's Like to Be a Child," For the Sake of Children [Special issue], *The New York Times Magazine,* October 8, 1995, p. 51.

2. Joy Overbeck, "Sex, Kids, and the Slut Look," *Newsweek,* July 26, 1993, p. 8.

3. Lucinda Franks, "Little Big People," *The New York Times Magazine,* October 10, 1993, p. 31.

4. Lawrence Zuckerman, "Out of the Mouth of Babes," *Time,* November 7, 1988.

5. Ellen Graham, "As Kids Gain the Power of the Purse, Marketing Takes Aim at Them," *The Wall Street Journal,* January 19, 1988.

6. Interview by Melissa Ludtke, *Time,* Special Issue: Through the Eyes of Children, August 8, 1988.

7. Emma Span, "This Is My Life," *Parenting,* December/January 1995, p. 108.

8. Letter from the Publisher, *Time,* Special Issue: Through the Eyes of Children, August 8, 1988.

9. Melissa Fay Greene, "Childhood Lost," *Parenting,* December/January 1995, p. 101.

10. Jules Feiffer, *This World, San Francisco Examiner,* September 20, 1992.

11. Theopia Jackson, Student Journal, Advanced Child Clinical Seminar, The Wright Institute, December 1993.

12. James Willwerth, "Hello, I'm Home Alone . . . ," *Time,* March 1, 1993.

13. "30% in Teen-Ager Survey Considered Suicide," *The New York Times,* September 14, 1988.

14. Carnegie Council on Adolescent Development, *Great Transitions,* October 1995.

15. Thomas M. Achenbach and Catherine T. Howell (1993), "Are American Children's Problems Getting Worse? A 13-Year Comparison," *Journal of the American Academy of Child and Adolescent Psychiatry,* Vol. 32, pp. 1145–1154.

16. Steve Waldman and Karen Springen, "Too Old, Too Fast?," *Newsweek,* November 16, 1992, p. 81.

17. Matthew Wald, "In New England Especially, Low Unemployment Spurs a New 'Child Labor,' " *The New York Times,* April 4, 1992, p. 7.

18. Quoted by Nell Bernstein as being found in the pages of *Mademoiselle* in Bernstein's article, "The No-Sale Generation," *San Francisco Examiner Image Magazine,* February 3, 1991, p. 6.

19. Results of poll cited in Jerry Carroll, "Young People Living in 'Prozac Nation,' " *San Francisco Chronicle,* September 28, 1994.

20. Jane Bryant Quinn, "The Luck of the Xers," *Newsweek,* June 6, 1994.

21. David M. Gross and Sophonia Scott, "Proceeding with Caution," *Time,* July 16, 1990, pp. 56–62.

22. Gregory Heller, Senior Class Speaker, the Thirty-First Commencement of Pitzer College, Claremont, California, May 14, 1995.

23. Quoted in David M. Gross and Sophonia Scott, op. cit., p. 58.

CHAPTER TEN

1. Penelope Leach (1994), *Children First,* New York: Alfred A. Knopf, p. 22.

2. Quoted in Gwen Kinkead, "Spock, Brazelton and Now . . . Penelope Leach," *The New York Times Magazine,* April 10, 1994, p. 54.

3. These findings were cited in Sue Shellenberger, Work and Family, "Moms and Dads Are the Scariest Monsters on Any Screen," *The Wall Street Journal,* October 26, 1994, p. 1.

4. Hillary Rodham Clinton (1996), *It Takes a Village,* New York, Simon and Schuster, p. 12.

• • •

5. See D. W. Winnicott (1963), "From Dependence towards Independence in the Development of the Individual," in *The Maturational Processes and the Facilitating Environment,* Madison, Connecticut: International Universities Press, pp. 83–92.

6. Barbara Vobejda, "Huge Majority of Day Care Centers Called Mediocre," *San Francisco Chronicle,* February 6, 1995, p. A3.

Index

Abuse. *See also* Child abuse
  verbal, toward parents, 75
Active listening, 169, 180
Adolescent(s). *See also* Kinder-
    dult(s)
  sense of identity in, 215, 217–
    218
  suicide of, 224
  work and, 144–145, 225–228
Adult(s). *See also* Father(s);
    Mother(s); Parent(s)
  young, dilemmas of, 228–230
Adultomorphic syndrome, 133
Aggression
  child's, 188–190
  in early childhood development,
    185–186
  guilt about, 188. *See also* Guilt
  integration of, 204
  parental, 182–183
    failure to acknowledge, 190–
      191
    positive versus negative percep-
      tions of, 186–187
  repression of, 187, 194–195
AIDS, telling children about, 17–18
Anger
  communicating with child about,
    188–189
  parental, 180–184

Anxiety
  separation, 153, 159–160, 173–
    174
  stranger, 153
  undoing, 115–120
Aries, Phillippe, 69
Attachment, theories of, 153
Attention deficit disorder, 105
Authority. *See also* Democracy
  defined, 193
  parental aversion to, 191–199,
    212–213
  social factors in, 198
Autonomy
  development of, 153–154
  drive for, 121

B

Barrie, James M., 12
Bedtime, timing of, 198
Behavior, ego syntonic versus ego
    dystonic, 86–87
Benjamin, Jessica, 49, 204–205
Bettelheim, Bruno, 2, 41, 46, 66
Birth, technology and, 30
Birth defects, parental response to,
    31–33
Bonds of Love, The, 49, 204–205

Boundaries
between adulthood and childhood, 67
demarcation of, 46–48
development of notion of, 49

C

Career. *See also* Work
balance between family life and,
82–83
parental, child's interests and,
63–68
Cheerleading, parental, 122–128
alternative to, 145–150
Child(ren). *See also* Adolescent(s);
Infant(s); Kinderdult(s)
advertising appeals to, 16
behavioral expectations for, 168–
169
as commodity, 25–29
decisions regarding custody of,
154–155
deification of, 127
demands for perfection of, 29–34
fears of, 10
and fears of rejection, 153–161
as friends versus dependents,
171, 178–179
gratification versus deprivation
of, 161–168
latchkey, 142–143, 224
material indulgence of, 166–168
overinvolvement with, 78
overprotection of, 128
overvaluing of, 23–25, 121–122
correcting, 42–45
parental expectations for, 33–34,
37–38
changing, 42
parents' bartering for love of,
151–177
as Pygmalion, 107–108
rejection of parents by, 156–157
resilience of, 238

respect for, 169
and response to parental stress,
233–234
self-aggrandizement of, 3–4
and sleeping with parents, 59–
61, 67–68
underdisciplined. *See also* Discipline
dangers for, 203–206
Child abuse
false reports of, 184–185
obligation to report, 184
Child development
alternative models of, 100–106
attachment to other human beings in, 153
at child's speed, 146
love and aggression in, 185–
186
mental health professionals' view
of, 105
play in, 130–131
Child rearing
as collective responsibility, 236–
237
economics as factor in, 56–57
self-esteem movement in, 122–
128
social factors in, 104–105
time-friendly work and, 235
by village, 234–241
Childhood
cultural concepts of, 13
essential, 130
loss of, 207–208
redefining, 13–18
unspoiling, 231–244
Children's rights, 155–156
Chodorow, Nancy, 72
Clegg, Hugh, 203
Clinton, Hillary Rodham, 33, 234
Clothes, child-adult boundaries
and, 68–71
Cognitive ability. *See also* Intellectual development
overemphasis of, 128–129
Combrinck-Graham, Lee, 197

Communication
   about anger, 188–189
   ineffective, 170–171
Corporal punishment
   prohibition of, 179–185
   during Puritan era, 183
Counseling, child in, 190
Creativity, play in development of,
   130–131
Culture. *See also* Society
   and concept of childhood, 13
Culture of Narcissism, The, 183
Custody, child, decisions regarding, 154–155

D

Deification, of children, 127
Democracy. *See also* Authority;
   Equality
   quest for, 169–172
Depression, parental, 52
Deprivation, versus gratification,
   161–168
Development
   child. *See* Child development
   intellectual, in infants and tod-
      dlers, 109–115
Difficult Child, The, 189
Disappointments, helping children
   with, 127–128
Discipline, 178–206. *See also*
   Limit setting
   and abnegation of adult author-
      ity, 191–199
   with corporal punishment, 179–185
   dangers of lack of, 203–206
   dispelling dangers of, 199–202
   love and aggression in, 185–191
   parental fears and, 185–191
Divorce
   decisions regarding child custody
      and, 154–156
   support for child of, 165–166
Dubroff, Jessica, 15

E

Economics, of child rearing, 56–57
Education, changing attitudes to-
   ward, 110–115
Ego, syntonic versus dystonic, 86–
   87
Elkind, David, 15, 41, 151
Elson, Miriam, 31
Emotions, of parents, 180–181
Equality. *See also* Authority; De-
   mocracy
   false notions of, 212–213
Expectations, parental, 93–120

F

Family(ies). *See also* Parent(s)
   versus career, 82–83
   child's role in, 140–145
   extended, absence of, 11
   fragile ties of, 10–11
   government intervention in, 155–
      156
   nuclear, in twenty-first century,
      242
   role reversal in, 154
   state of flux in, 5–7
Father(s). *See also* Parent(s)
   children as extension of, 72–73
Fear
   of children, 221–222
   parental, 185–191
Feiffer, Jules, 222
Fetus
   screening for genetic anomalies
      in, 30, 32
   stimulation of, 108–109
Fitzpatrick, Jean, 129
Flex-time, 235
Franks, Lucinda, 54, 208
Free schools, 162–163
Freud, Sigmund, 23, 24, 36, 50
   on deprivation, 162
Friends, imaginary, 216

G

Generation X, 228
Genetic anomalies, screening for,
    30, 32
Goleman, Daniel, 169
Gordon, Thomas, 180
Gratification, versus deprivation,
    161–168
Guilt, 74–92, 106
    about parental aggression, 188
    about physically punishing child,
        182
    definition of, 74
    and kinderdult, 89–92
    and overindulgence of child, 81
    parental, 34, 39
    parenting by, 239–240
    and parenting by beeper, 88–89
    from physically punishing child,
        179–180
    and pursuit of happiness, 86–87
    recognizing, 80
    undoing, 115–120
    and vacillation between overin-
        dulgence and neglect, 91–92
    work as external factor in, 81–82

H

Healing, parental, 42–45, 115–120
Hewlett, Sylvia, 65
Hitting. See also Corporal punish-
    ment
    prohibition of, 179–185
Homework, parental involvement
    in, 76, 79, 84, 135–137
Hurried Child, The, 15

I

Identity. See also Self
    of adolescent, 215, 217–218
    development of, 215

kinderdult's confusion about,
        214–218
    split, 217
Imaginary friends, 216
Individual, cultural emphasis on,
    48–50
Infant(s). See also Child(ren)
    accommodating of parents by,
        51–52
    autonomy of, 153–154
    intellectual stimulation of, 109,
        132
Intellectual development. See also
    Cognitive ability
    in infants and toddlers, 109–
        115
    premature emphasis on, 132
    stress due to, 114
Intimacy, sexual, after birth of
    child, 60–61

K

Kahn, Alice, 12–13
Kinderdult(s), 17–18, 207–230.
    See also Adolescent(s);
    Child(ren)
    adolescent, work and, 225–228
    assets of, 210
    and attitudes toward future, 228–
        230
    confused identity of, 214–218
    and confusion between gratifica-
        tion and deprivation, 168
    desires of, 218–221
    internal conflicts of, 214–225
    internal safety of, 221–225
    interview with, 211–214
    parental guilt and, 89–92
    as parents, 220
    risks of, 210–211
Kindergarten readiness movement,
    113
Kingsley, Gregory, 155
Kohut, Heinz, 48

L

La Leche League, 59
Lasch, Christopher, 183, 193–194
Latchkey children, 142–143, 224
Leach, Penelope, 231, 232
Libido, in child development, 185–
186
Limit setting. *See also* Discipline
absence of, 162–165
children's desire for, 220
difficulty with, 178
Listening
active, 169, 180
pros and cons of, 169
Lord of the Flies, The, 163
Love
bartering for
basic tenets of, 153
ending practice of, 240–241
false independence as result of,
172–177
gratification versus deprivation
in, 161–168
respect versus overindulgence
in, 168–172
as commodity, 156
and gratification of children,
163–168
in human development, 185–186
parents' bartering for, 151–177
versus respect, 152
"tough," 158
Ludtke, Melissa, 217, 220

M

Mahler, Margaret, 48
Marriage, changing status of, 10–
11
Materialism, 166–168
Mental illness, blaming parents
for, 104–105
Miller, Alice, 107
Mirroring, 50–55

Montessori, Maria, 129
Mother(s). *See also* Parent(s)
blaming, for mental disorders,
105
children as extension of, 72–73
working, 2–3
working versus stay-at-home,
161–162

N

Narcissism, parental, 34–42, 119
healing, 42–45
Native American culture, training
of children in, 139–140
Nature versus nurture controversy,
100–106

O

Overworked American, The, 81–82

P

Parent(s). *See also* Family(ies); Father(s); Mother(s)
blaming, 104–105
changing society's treatment of,
235–236
child sleeping with, 59–61, 67–68
confusion of, 4–7
insight into, 19–22
demands for perfection by, 29–34
expectation for perfection of,
238–239
expectations of, 93–120
and fear of child's rejection, 153–
161, 156–158
fears of, 185–191
guilt of, 239–240
interests of, versus child's interests, 63–68
narcissism of, 35–42

Parent(s) *(continued)*
and need to be liked by children, 151
needs of, versus baby's, 46
overinvolvement of, with children, 78
pressures on, 231–233
pushy, 110–115
reducing stress of, 233–234
respect versus love for, 152
self-centered, 2. *See also* Narcissism; Self-centeredness
stress of, 235
underaggressive, 187–188
undoing anxiety, guilt, and pushiness of, 115–120
Parent Effectiveness Training, 180–181
Parenthood
delayed, 27–28
inevitable versus chosen, 57
love and aggression and, 185
as marker of adulthood, 47
Parenting
available time for, 8–9
by beeper, 88–89
crisis of, 5
economic considerations in, 56–57
and fear for children's future, 9–10
by guilt. *See* Guilt
historical perspective on, 6
"just due" versus "just do," 240–241
paradox of, 2–4
perils of, 1–22
and Peter Pan syndrome, 11–13
redefining, 13–18
structural aspects of, 8–13
in twenty-first century, 242–244
Perfection, expectations about, 238–239
Permissiveness
and repression of aggression, 187
trend toward, 162–168
Personality, components of, 186

Peter Pan syndrome, 11–13, 228
discipline and, 191–192
Play
developing capacity for, 148
disappearance of, 128–135
incapacity for, 132–133
value of, 130–131
Problems, parental fixing of, 127–128
Punishment, corporal
prohibition of, 179–185
during Puritan era, 183
Pygmalion, child as, 107–108

Q

Quindlen, Anna, 58

R

Ramey, Craig, 109
Rejection, children's and parents' fears of, 153–161
Reparative Motif, The, 203
Respect
for children, 169
of children, 169
versus love, 152
Rewards, for building self-esteem, 123
Ryan, Joan, 21

S

Safety, children's concerns about, 221–225
Samalin, Barbara, 178
Schools. *See also* Education
free, 162–163
Schor, Juliet, 81–83
Self. *See also* Identity
definition of, 217–218
development of, 48–50

false, development of, 145–147
true, 186
Self-centeredness. *See also* Narcissism
parental, 2–4, 81
Self-esteem
versus actual performance, 124
child's, 122
Self-esteem movement, 122–128
alternative to, 126, 145–150
purpose of, 123–124
Separation anxiety, 153, 159–160,
173–174
Sexual intimacy, after birth of
child, 60–61
Sexuality, precocious, 207
Skinner, B.F., 100
Social angst, 41
Society
changing priorities and practices
of, 235–236
child rearing and, 234–241
as factor in child rearing, 104–105
Sonic belt, 108–109
Spock, Benjamin, 6, 59, 121, 187, 193
Stern, Daniel, 48–49
Stevenson, Harold, 124
Stranger anxiety, 153
Stress, parental, 235
reducing, 233–234
Success, pushing children toward,
121–150
remedies for, 145–150
symptoms of child's resistance
to, 146–147
Suicide, teenage, 224
Summerhill, 162
Superbaby Syndrome, The, 129

T

Taffel, Ronald, 163
Technology, birth, and demands
for perfection of infants, 30, 32
Teenager. *See* Adolescent(s); Kinder-
dult(s)

Therapy, child in, 190
Time
availability of, 8–9
quality, 9, 79, 84
Too Precious Child, The, 56
Tough Love programs, 158
Toys, educational, 109
Twin studies, 103–104

V

Village, child raising by, 234–241
Violence
fears of, 221–222
increasing incidence of, 183

W

Watson, John B., 100
*When the Bough Breaks: The Cost
of Neglecting Our Children,* 65
Winnicott, D.W., 48, 50, 140,
187, 203, 238
Work. *See also* Career
adolescent kinderdult and, 225–
228
children's, in traditional versus
U.S. culture, 140–145
educational preparation and,
228–230
effect of, on parenting, 8–9
as external factor in parental
guilt, 81–82
mothers' anxieties about, 161–
162
parental, child's interests and,
63–68
time-friendly, 235

Y

Young adult(s), dilemmas of, 228–
230